Manual of Medical Treatment in Urology

Manual of Medical Treatment in Urology

Editors

Ismaila A Mungadi MBBS FRCS(Edin) FWACS FMAS
Professor of Surgery/Consultant Urologist
Usmanu Danfodiyo University and
Usmanu Danfodiyo University Teaching Hospital
Sokoto, Nigeria

(Late) Hyacinth N Mbibu MBBS BSc FWACS
Professor of Urology
Ahmadu Bello University and
Ahmadu Bello University Teaching Hospital
Zaria, Nigeria

Ehab Eltahawy MD MRCS
Assistant Professor of Urology
Division of Reconstructive and Endourology
University of Arkansas for Medical Sciences
W Markham, USA

Abdullahi Abdulwahab-Ahmed MBBS FMCS
Senior Lecturer/Consultant Urologist
Usmanu Danfodiyo University and
Usmanu Danfodiyo University Teaching Hospital
Sokoto, Nigeria

Foreword
Y Ahmed

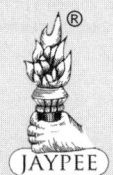

JAYPEE BROTHERS MEDICAL PUBLISHERS (P) LTD
New Delhi • London • Philadelphia • Panama

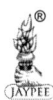 **Jaypee Brothers Medical Publishers (P) Ltd**

Headquarters

Jaypee Brothers Medical Publishers (P) Ltd
4838/24, Ansari Road, Daryaganj
New Delhi 110 002, India
Phone: +91-11-43574357
Fax: +91-11-43574314
Email: jaypee@jaypeebrothers.com

Overseas Offices

J.P. Medical Ltd
83, Victoria Street, London
SW1H 0HW (UK)
Phone: +44-2031708910
Fax: +02-03-0086180
Email: info@jpmedpub.com

Jaypee-Highlights
Medical Publishers Inc.
City of Knowledge, Bld. 237
Clayton, Panama City, Panama
Phone: +507-301-0496
Fax: +507-301-0499
Email: cservice@jphmedical.com

Jaypee Medical Inc.
The Bourse
111 South Independence Mall East
Suite 835, Philadelphia, PA 19106, USA
Phone: + 267-519-9789
Email: jpmed.us@gmail.com

Jaypee Brothers
Medical Publishers (P) Ltd
17/1-B Babar Road, Block-B
Shaymali, Mohammadpur
Dhaka-1207, Bangladesh
Mobile: +08801912003485
Email: jaypeedhaka@gmail.com

Jaypee Brothers
Medical Publishers (P) Ltd
Shorakhute, Kathmandu
Nepal
Phone: +00977-9841528578
Email: jaypee.nepal@gmail.com

Website: www.jaypeebrothers.com
Website: www.jaypeedigital.com

© 2014, Jaypee Brothers Medical Publishers

All rights reserved. No part of this book may be reproduced in any form or by any means without the prior permission of the publisher.

Inquiries for bulk sales may be solicited at: jaypee@jaypeebrothers.com

This book has been published in good faith that the contents provided by the contributors contained herein are original, and is intended for educational purposes only. While every effort is made to ensure accuracy of information, the publisher and the editors specifically disclaim any damage, liability, or loss incurred, directly or indirectly, from the use or application of any of the contents of this work. If not specifically stated, all figures and tables are courtesy of the editors. Where appropriate, the readers should consult with a specialist or contact the manufacturer of the drug or device.

Manual of Medical Treatment in Urology

First Edition: **2014**

ISBN: 978-93-5090-844-0

Printed at Rajkamal Electric Press, Plot No. 2, Phase-IV, Kundli, Haryana.

Dedicated to

*The memory of (late) Hyacinth N Mbibu, professor of Urology.
His demise to the bullet of unknown assailants occurred a few days after
signing the publication agreement of this book.*

Contributors

Aliu Abdulhameed MBBS
Department of Surgery
Usmanu Danfodiyo University
Teaching Hospital, Sokoto, Nigeria

Abdullahi Abdulwahab-Ahmed MBBS FMCS
Senior Lecturer/Consultant Urologist
Usmanu Danfodiyo University and
Usmanu Danfodiyo University
Teaching Hospital
Sokoto, Nigeria

Emmanuel A Ameh MBBS FWACS FACS
Professor of Pediatric Surgery
Chief, Division of Pediatric Surgery
Department of Surgery
Ahmadu Bello University and
Ahmadu Bello University Teaching
Hospital, Zaria, Nigeria

Ngwobia P Agwu MBBS FMCS
Consultant Urologist
Department of Surgery
Usmanu Danfodiyo University
Teaching Hospital
Sokoto, Nigeria

Ehab Eltahawy MD MRCS
Assistant Professor of Urology
Division of Reconstructive and
Endourology
University of Arkansas for
Medical Sciences
W Markham, USA

Stella A Eguma MBBS DA FWACS
Professor of Anesthesia
Ahmadu Bello University
Consultant Anesthetist
Ahmadu Bello University
Teaching Hospital, Zaria, Nigeria
Consultant Anesthesiologist/Director
Nurse Anesthesia Training Program
John F Kennedy Memorial Hospital
Monrovia, Liberia

Samy Heshmat MD
Urology Resident
University of Arkansas for
Medical Sciences, W Markham, USA

Mohamed H Kamel MD
Assistant Professor of Urology
Uro-Oncology and Robotic
Uro-Surgery
University of Arkansas for Medical
Sciences, W Markham, USA

Hamidu M Liman MBBS FMCP
Lecturer/Consultant Nephrologist
Department of Medicine
Usmanu Danfodiyo University and
Usmanu Danfodiyo University
Teaching Hospital, Sokoto, Nigeria

Christopher S Lukong MBBS FWACS
Senior Lecturer/ Consultant Pediatric
Surgeon
Department of Surgery
Usmanu Danfodiyo University and
Usmanu Danfodiyo University
Teaching Hospital, Sokoto, Nigeria

Ayman Mahdy MD
Assistant Professor
Department of Urology
The University of Arkansas for
Medical Sciences, W Markham, USA

(Late) Hyacinth N Mbibu MBBS BSc FWACS
Professor of Urology
Ahmadu Bello University and
Ahmadu Bello University Teaching
Hospital, Zaria, Nigeria

Ismaila A Mungadi MBBS FRCS(Edin) FWACS FMAS
Professor of Surgery/Consultant
Urologist, Usmanu Danfodiyo
University and Usmanu Danfodiyo
University Teaching Hospital
Sokoto, Nigeria

Abdulkadir A Salako MBBS FWACS
Senior Lecturer/Consultant Urologist
Department of Surgery
Obafemi Awolowo University and
Obafemi Awolowo University
Teaching Hospital Complex
Ile-Ife, Nigeria

Olayiwola B Shittu MBBS FRCS FWACS
Professor of Urology
Department of Surgery
University College Hospital
Ibadan, Nigeria

Foreword

The management of urological diseases has undergone drastic changes over the years. With the successful management of BPH and LUTS using drugs, there has been an increasing role of drug treatment in urological practice. Effective drug therapy is now known for the management of erectile dysfunction and overactive bladder. Medical treatment is an integral component of urological practice. This trend is not limited only to benign urological conditions; there has been scientific research for an effective and tolerable drug treatment for urological cancers. This has witnessed the introduction of agents for the treatment of most urological cancers.

Giving the increasing role of drugs use in urological practice, the need for a manual of medical treatment in urology cannot be overemphasized. The manual is timely, and aids the surgical residents, urology residents, practicing urologists and general practitioners in keeping pace with this new and rapidly expanding field of urology.

The authors have gone to a great extent to organize this unique book into easily readable chapters with an outline of the drugs following each chapter. This arrangement guides the reader and serves as a quick office reference on prescription. The editors and authors have done a commendable work. However, they need to revise the book regularly.

Y Ahmed MBBS FWACS
Chief Medical Director
Usmanu Danfodiyo University
Teaching Hospital
Sokoto, Nigeria

Preface

There are a large number of books published every year on the surgical aspects of urology. As urologists and patients get more interested in minimally and less invasive options for their diseases, we were motivated to prepare a book on the different aspects of medical care for urological diseases. This book will help the general urologist to identify the recent trends in the medical management and act as a guide to the office practice of such conditions.

The existence of many urological diseases that can be treated or palliated medically, call for succinct manual to the medical treatment of such conditions. Most urological infections are primarily treated medically, unless complicated. Some conditions that are usually treated medically include erectile dysfunction, pain syndromes and bladder overactivity. In another group of urological diseases, medical treatment may be the initial rational therapy in many situations and many patients tend to be inclined to this. A good example can be found in the treatment of lower urinary tract symptoms secondary to benign prostatic enlargement. In urological cancers, medical therapy is an integral part of treatment or palliation depending on histological type, grade and stage of malignancy.

This book will guide readers on the choice of medical therapy for various urological conditions, and will provide handy office reference on drug choice, complications and dosing. Drug therapy is a very dynamic area and readers are advised to verify pharmacotherapeutic information from current evidence-based protocols and manufacturers' guide.

Ismaila A Mungadi
(Late) Hyacinth N Mbibu
Ehab Eltahawy
Abdullahi Abdulwahab-Ahmed

Acknowledgments

We appreciate the contribution of M/s Jaypee Brothers Medical Publishers (P) Ltd., New Delhi, India, in making this project a success. In particular mention are Ms Chetna Malhotra Vohra (Senior Manager–Business Development) for her belief in our group's ability to deliver and Ms Saima Rashid (Development Editor) who did very well in making sure we catch up with the deadline.

Contents

Section 1: Benign Urological Diseases

1. **Medical Treatment of Pain** — 3
   Ismaila A Mungadi, Stella A Eguma, Abdullahi Abdulwahab-Ahmed
   - Pain Assessment — 4
   - Renal and Ureteric Colic — 5
   - Chronic Pelvic Pain Syndrome (CPPS) — 5
   - Interstitial Cystitis — 6
   - Urological Cancer Pain — 6
   - Postoperative Analgesia — 6
   - Outline of Pharmacotherapy — 7

2. **Antimicrobial Therapy** — 13
   Ismaila A Mungadi, Hamidu M Liman, Aliu Abdulhameed
   - General Principles and Guidelines to Therapy — 13
   - Acute Pyelonephritis — 14
   - Cystitis — 15
   - Bacterial Prostatitis — 15
   - Epididymitis, Epididymo-orchitis — 16
   - Genitourinary Tuberculosis — 16
   - Urethritis — 17
   - Syphilis and Other Sexually Transmitted Infections — 17
   - Genital Herpes — 18
   - Molluscum Contagiosum — 18
   - Urinary Schistosomiasis — 18
   - Scrotal Filariasis — 18
   - Fungal Infection — 19
   - Actinomycosis — 20
   - Fournier's Gangrene — 20
   - Perioperative Antimicrobial Prophylaxis — 21
   - Outline of Pharmacotherapy — 22

3. **Medical Management of Erectile Dysfunction** — 40
   Samy Heshmat, Ehab Eltahawy
   - Patient Evaluation — 40
   - Treatment of Erectile Dysfunction — 42
   - Outline of Pharmacologic Therapy — 44

4. **Medical Treatment of Urinary Incontinence** 51
   Ayman Mahdy, Ismaila A Mungadi
   - Control of Micturition 51
   - Evaluation of Urinary Incontinence Patients 52
   - How Can We Prevent Urinary Incontinence? 52
   - Urinary Incontinence Management Options 53
   - Role of Pharmacotherapy 54
   - Outline of Some Pharmacotherapeutic Agents 57

5. **Benign Prostatic Hyperplasia** 62
   Ismaila A Mungadi, Olayiwola B Shittu, Abdullahi Abdulwahab-Ahmed
   - Alpha-Adrenergic Antagonist 63
   - 5-alpha Reductase Inhibitors 63
   - Combination Therapy 65
   - Phytotherapeutic Agents 65
   - Outline of Pharmacotherapy for BPH 66

6. **Medical Treatment of Urolithiasis** 71
   Ehab Eltahawy, Ismaila A Mungadi
   - Risk Stratification 71
   - Evaluation of Nephrolithiasis 72
   - Medical Therapy 74
   - Follow-up Studies 79

7. **Miscellaneous Use of Drugs** 82
   (Late) Hyacinth N Mbibu, Ismaila A Mungadi
   - Premature Ejaculation 82
   - Priapism 82
   - Infertility 84

Section 2: Medical Treatment of Urological Cancer

8. **Renal Cell Carcinoma** 89
   Ismaila A Mungadi, (Late) Hyacinth N Mbibu, Abdullahi Abdulwahab-Ahmed
   - Drug Treatment of RCC 89
   - Outline of Pharmacotherapy 91

9. **Bladder Cancer** 94
   Ismaila A Mungadi, Mohamed H Kamel, Ngwobia P Agwu
   - Intravesical Therapy for Superficial Bladder Cancer 96
   - Intravesical Immunotherapy 96
   - Intravesical Chemotherapy 99

• Photodynamic Therapy	99
• Combination Therapy and Timing	99
• Invasive Bladder Cancer	99
• Systemic Chemotherapy for Metastatic Disease	100
• Other Guidelines	101
• Details of Pharmacotherapy for Bladder Cancer	102

10. Prostate Cancer — 113
Ismaila A Mungadi, Olayiwola B Shittu, Abdullahi Abdulwahab-Ahmed

- Role of Medical Treatment — 113
- Outline of Pharmacotherapy for Prostate Cancer — 116

11. Testicular Cancer — 125
Ismaila A Mungadi, Abdulkadir A Salako

- Diagnosis and Staging of Germ Cell Tumor — 125
- Role of Tumor Marker — 127
- Role of Chemotherapy in the Treatment of Testicular Tumor — 129
- Outline of Pharmacotherapy — 132

12. Squamous Cell Carcinoma of the Penis — 137
Ismaila A Mungadi, Abdullahi Abdulwahab-Ahmed

- Treatment of Penile Cancer — 138
- Outline of Drug for Treatment of Penile Cancer — 140

13. Nephroblastoma (Wilms' Tumor) — 142
Christopher S Lukong, Emmanuel A Ameh

- Staging — 143
- Tumor Grading — 143
- Principles of Treatment and Treatment Modalities — 144

Appendix

Normal Values of Some Laboratory Tests of Urological Interest — 151

- Biochemical — 151
- Hematological — 153
- Hormones — 153
- Renal Function — 154

Index — *157*

Plate 1

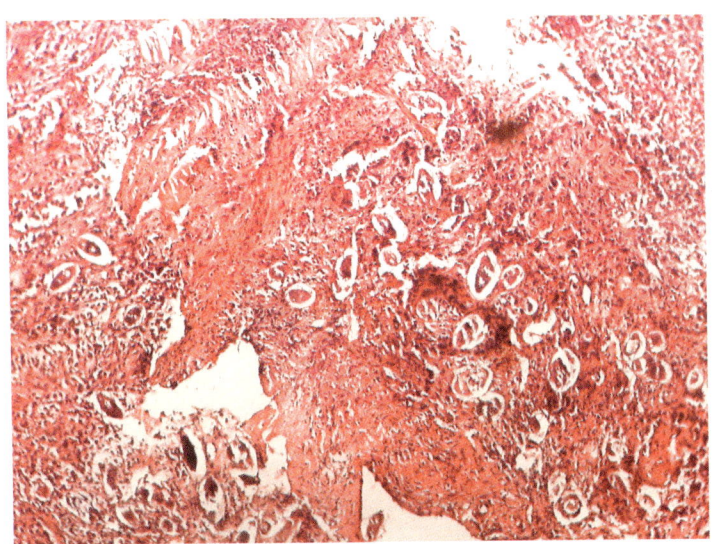

Fig. 2.1: Calcified ova of *Schistosoma haematobium* associated with bladder carcinoma

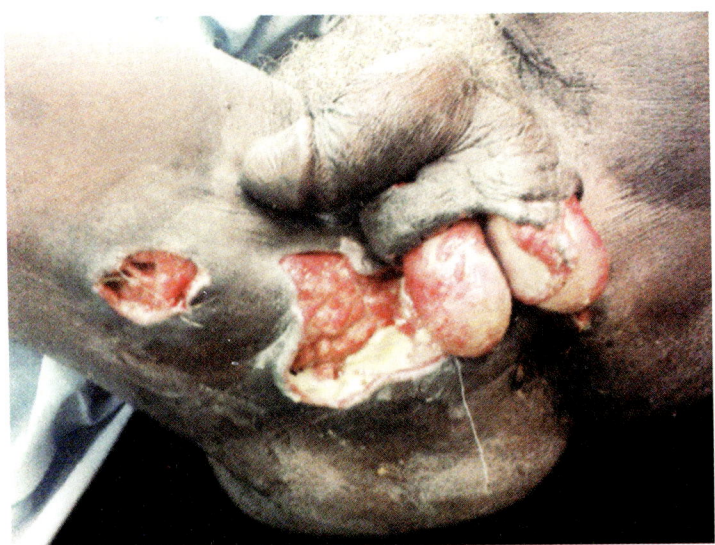

Fig. 2.2: Fournier's gangrene

Plate 2

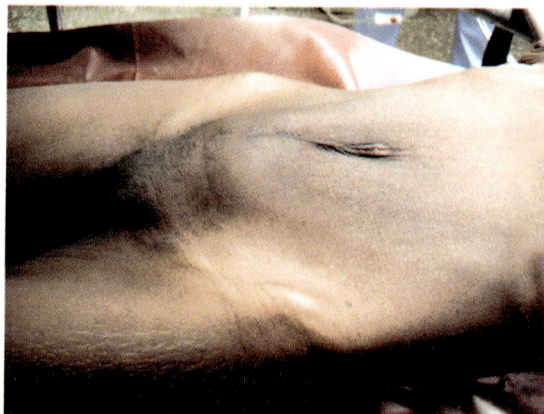

Fig. 9.1: A lady with advanced bladder carcinoma

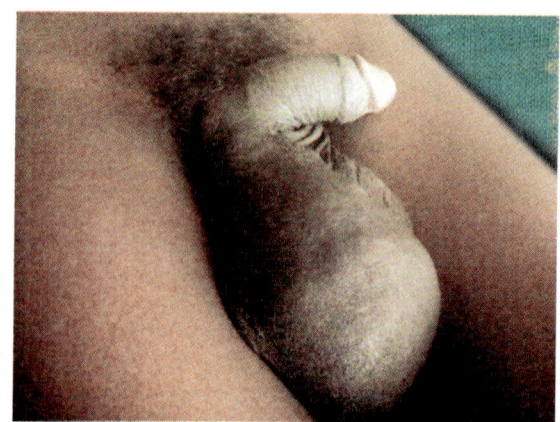

Fig. 11.1: Early testicular tumor in a 24-year old boy with gynecomastia

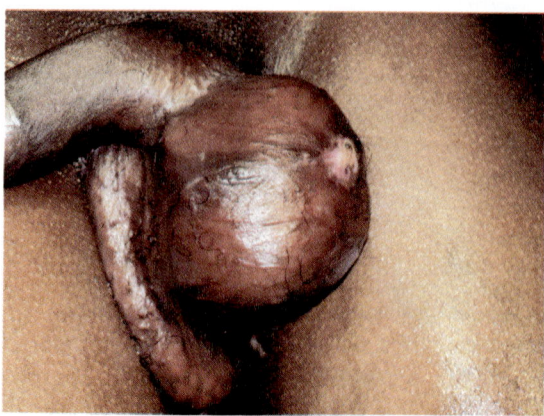

Fig. 11.2: Locally advanced testicular tumor

Plate 3

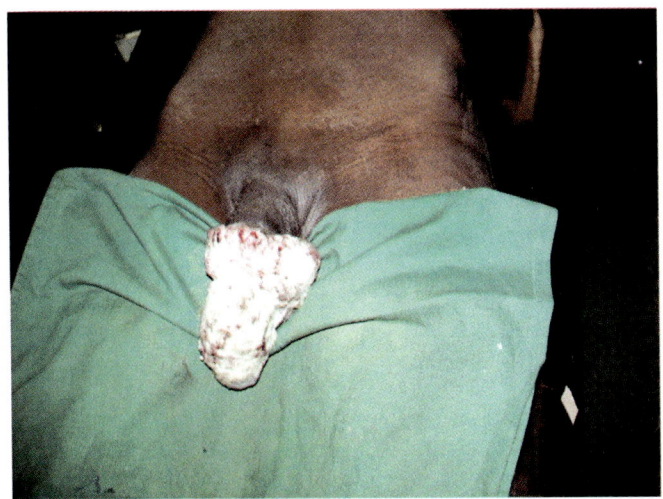

Fig. 12.1: Late penile cancer

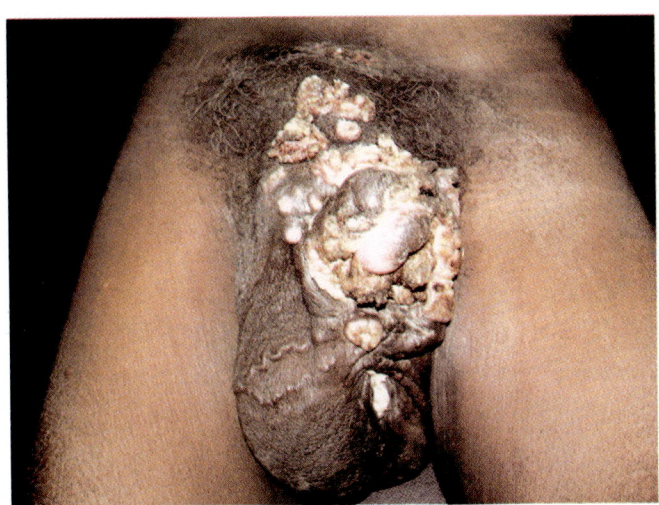

Fig. 12.2: Very late penile cancer

SECTION 1

BENIGN UROLOGICAL DISEASES

Medical Treatment of Pain
Ismaila A Mungadi, Stella A Eguma, Abdullahi Abdulwahab-Ahmed

Antimicrobial Therapy
Ismaila A Mungadi, Hamidu M Liman, Aliu Abdulhameed

Medical Management of Erectile Dysfunction
Samy Heshmat, Ehab Eltahawy

Medical Treatment of Urinary Incontinence
Ayman Mahdy, Ismaila A Mungadi

Benign Prostatic Hyperplasia
Ismaila A Mungadi, Olayiwola B Shittu, Abdullahi Abdulwahab-Ahmed

Medical Treatment of Urolithiasis
Ehab Eltahawy, Ismaila A Mungadi

Miscellaneous Use of Drugs
(Late) Hyacinth N Mbibu, Ismaila A Mungadi

CHAPTER 1

Medical Treatment of Pain

Ismaila A Mungadi, Stella A Eguma, Abdullahi Abdulwahab-Ahmed

■ INTRODUCTION

Pain is an unpleasant sensory and emotional experience associated with actual or potential tissue damage or described in terms of such damage.[1,2]

Urologic pain may be local, originating from the organ itself or be referred from surrounding diseased organs. Due to common innervations, urologic pain is often referred to other sites, and so gastroenteric and gynecological pain may indeed signify urologic pathology.

Pain in the urinary tract may result from distension, inflammation, carcinoma, ischemia, or infection of the urinary tract. The severity of pain varies depending on the onset of the cause of pain. Noxious stimuli from the urinary tract are transmitted via A-delta and C fibers to the spinal cord through the dorsal roots. There, they synapse on neurons within the dorsal horn of the spinal cord segment that they entered and also on neurons one to two segments above and below their segment of entry. The secondary neurons ascend through the spinothalamic tract through the medulla and synapse on neurons in the thalamus. Some neurons also synapse in the medulla's reticular formation. Nerves from the thalamus then relay the signal to the somatosensory cortex where the stimulus is interpreted as pain (Fig. 1.1).

In addition, when tissue is damaged or there is a noxious pathological stimulus, second messenger systems are activated resulting in the release of inflammatory mediators (bradykinin, histamine, prostaglandins, serotonin) at the site of injury, and this results in pain produced by tissue damage or by pathological processes.

The management of most urologic pains should proceed according to the analgesic ladder proposed by the World Health Organization (WHO) (Fig. 1.2).[3] This is applicable to cancer pain and management of prostatitis and chronic pelvic pain syndromes. The starting dosage should be individualized paying attention to patient age, preexisting diseases and other risk factors.

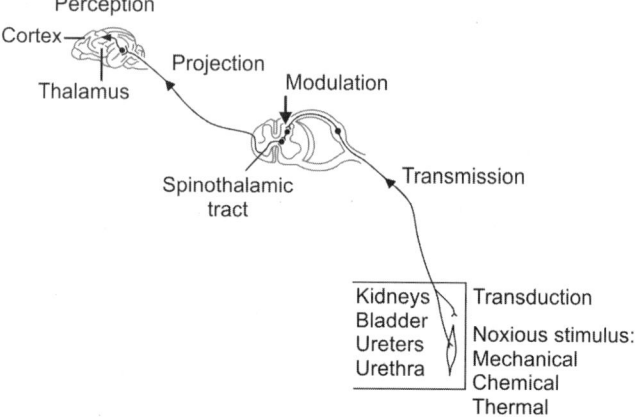

Fig. 1.1: Pain pathway

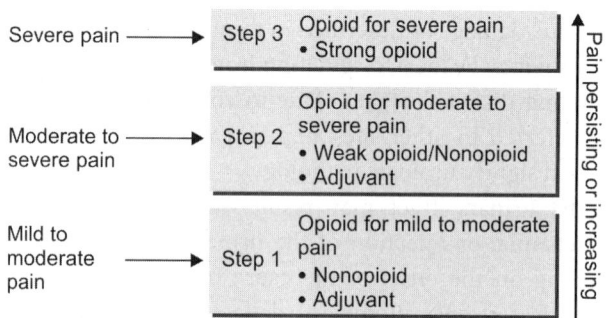

Fig. 1.2: WHO analgesic ladder

PAIN ASSESSMENT

For effective management, pain should be measured. This facilitates assessment of efficacy of medical treatment and allows comparison of treatment modalities employed. Various grading systems exist. There is no absolute measurement of the degree of pain. Pain is subjective. Numerical rating scales ask patients to judge their pain intensity on a scale from 0 (no pain at all) to 10 (unimaginable pain). Other assessment scales include visual analog scales (VAS), numeric pain intensity scale, verbal rating scale, and pain faces scale (used for children over 5 years), and the McGill Pain Questionnaire.

Visual Analogue Scale

A visual analogue scale is a measurement instrument that tries to measure the amount of pain that a patient feels across a continuum from none to an extreme amount of pain. It is usually a horizontal line, 100 mm in length and marked with "no pain" at one end and "very severe pain" at the other end. The patient marks on the line the point that they feel represents their perception of their pain. The VAS score is determined by measuring in millimeters from the left-hand end of the line to the point that the patient marks.

No pain_____ Very severe pain

■ RENAL AND URETERIC COLIC

Renal and ureteric colic results from increased pressure and tension in the renal pelvis and ureter secondary to obstruction. Renal inflammation leads to increased accumulation of pain mediators that can also increase blood flow and enhance urine production thus exacerbating the pain. Both nonsteroidal anti-inflammatory drugs (NSAIDs) and opioids are effective. NSAIDs also reduce renal blood flow and urine production thus reducing pressure and tension proximal to obstruction. Drugs with ureteric spasmolytic effect may be used as adjuvants in the treatment of ureteric colic. Drugs that may have adjuvant role in ureteric colic but are not in routine clinical practice include muscarinic agonists, desmopressin, nitrites, and calcium channel blockers. The use of alpha-adrenergic blockers (e.g. Tamsulosin) or calcium channel blockers (e.g. Nifedipine) may reduce pain and improve spontaneous passage of ureteric stones.[4]

■ CHRONIC PELVIC PAIN SYNDROME (CPPS)

This chronic nonbacterial prostatitis is one of the most difficult conditions to treat. It presents with genitourinary pain in the absence of identifiable uropathogenic bacteria. Pain is localized to the perineum, penis, or suprapubic area. This may be associated with testicular, perineal, anal, suprapubic, and rectal pain. There may be discomfort when sitting, post bowel movement pain, low back pain, or ejaculatory pain. Urinary frequency, urgency, hesitancy, burning, frequent night-time urination, and post-orgasm discomfort (often the next day) may occur. There may be related dyssynergic voiding and intraprostatic ductal reflux. A feeling of anxiety, depression, and helplessness often sets in.

There is no standardized evidence-based drug therapy for CPPS. At present a combination of antibiotics, anti-inflammatory drugs, adrenergic blockers, muscle relaxants, antidepressants, benzodiazepine, and finasteride can be tried. Also sitz baths and biofeedback techniques may offer some relief. When the pain is exacerbated by ingestion of certain substances like alcohol, caffeine, and some foodstuff, dietary restriction is recommended. Adrenergic blockers are more appropriate in patients with urodynamic evidence of outflow obstruction. Pentosan polysulphate may be tried in patients with interstitial cystitis–like symptoms.[5]

■ INTERSTITIAL CYSTITIS

Interstitial cystitis is a chronic pelvic pain syndrome that affects men and women of all cultures, socioeconomic backgrounds, and ages. The pathology reveals a damaged urinary tract endothelium. The etiology is unknown; however, sensory nervous system abnormalities, autoimmunity, and increased urothelial permeability are the main theories of causation of interstitial cystitis. The pain of interstitial cystitis is worsened with bladder filling and improved with urination. Certain foods or drink may worsen the pain.

There may be pain with sexual intercourse, and discomfort and difficulty while driving, travelling, or working.

Treatment of interstitial cystitis pain is also empirical. Therapy is typically multimodal, including the use of a bladder coating, an antihistamine to help control mast cell activity, and a low dose antidepressant to fight neurogenic inflammation. Intravesical instillation of pentosan polysulfate sodium,[5] dimethylsulphoxide, and BTX-A may help in nonoral medication responders. The use of a variety of traditional pain medications, including opiates and synthetic opioids such as tramadol, is often necessary to treat the varying degrees of pain.

■ UROLOGICAL CANCER PAIN

Cancer-related pain can be very incapacitating. The aim of drug therapy is to palliate the symptoms and improve the quality of life. The recommendation of the WHO expert committee on cancer pain relief has been validated. The committee recommends round-the-clock and oral therapy whenever possible. Treatment should progress according to the analgesic ladder (Fig. 1.2) and be tailored toward individual needs.

Adjuvant therapy varies depending on the cancer, the stage, and site of involvement and the type of metastasis. Bone metastasis in patients with prostatic cancer may require treatment with calcitonin, biphosphonate (pamidronate, ibandronate, zoledronic acid), or corticosteroids in addition of conventional analgesics.

Neuropathic pain may respond to tricyclic antidepressant and anticonvulsants (Carbamazepine, Phenytoin, Valproate, Clonazepam, Gabapentin) in addition to analgesics. Visceral pain may be alleviated with Octereotide or Oxybutinin.

■ POSTOPERATIVE ANALGESIA

A clear understanding of postoperative pain is essential for effective control. Postoperative pain is a type of acute pain and is a manifestation of autonomic, psychological, and behavioral responses to surgical trauma that result in an unpleasant, sensory, and emotional experience. Following surgery, the trauma triggers neurohumoral responses to facilitate healing as well as release of local response mediators that lead to pain. Treatment of pain is essential because inadequately managed pain may exacerbate patient discomfort and dissatisfaction, prolong hospital stay, prompt undue medical expense, and result in poor surgical outcome.

The goal for postoperative pain management is to reduce or eliminate pain and discomfort with a minimum of side effects at low cost.

Analgesia should be started promptly and given regularly. A stepwise approach is advocated depending on the severity of pain. If oral dosing has to be delayed, then initial intravenous, epidural, or intrathecal route may be resorted to. Rectal, buccal, or sublingual route, where appropriate, can be very valuable and these routes avoid first-pass metabolism. Local anesthetics provide effective relief and can be used topically; by infiltration, by wound irrigation or nerve blockade.

NSAIDs are particularly effective in postoperative pain because the associated inflammation sensitizes pain fibers. In our experience, a combination of paracetamol and a nonsteroidal anti-inflammatory drugs will control majority of postoperative pains, except in severe cases. This is also effective for most day-care surgery.

■ OUTLINE OF PHARMACOTHERAPY[6,7]

Nonopioids

Paracetamol (Acetaminophen)

Mechanism: Centrally acting antipyretic and analgesic. Precise mechanism unknown.

Indication: Mild to moderate pain.

Side effects: Hypersensitivity, hepatotoxicity, renal damage, contact dermatitis (injectable).

Precaution: Renal and hepatic impairment.

Interactions: Coumarins (enhances coumarins), cholestyramine (reduces absorption of paracetamol), metoclopramide, and domperidone (enhances absorption of paracetamol).

Dosage: 0.5–1 g four times a day, children 90 mg/kg/day in divided doses.

Preparations: Oral, injectable (proparacetamol)

Nonsteroidal Anti-inflammatory Drugs

Mechanism: Inhibit prostaglandin synthesis at therapeutic doses.

Indication: Mild to moderate inflammatory and postoperative pain. Renal and ureteric colic.

Shared side effects: Gastrointestinal symptoms including ulceration, hemorrhage, perforation, renal impairment, fluid retention, hypersensitivity, headaches, premature closure of ductus arteriosus, and inhibition of labor.

Contraindications: Active peptic ulcer, hypersensitivity, renal impairment, pregnancy.

Precaution: Allergic disorders, coagulation defects.

Interactions: Angiotensin-converting enzyme inhibitor (ACE; antagonism), other NSAIDs (increased side effects), antacids (absorption reduced), anticoagulants (enhanced anticoagulant activity) antihypertensive (enhanced hypertensive effects), diuretic (increased risk of nephrotoxicity). Other drugs that may interact with NSAIDs are antidepressants, cardiac glycosides, methotrexate, nitrates, phenytoin, sulphonylureas, corticosteroids, lithium, rifampicin, ketoconazole, haloperidol, zidovudine, biphosphates, cyclosporins, estrogens, progestogens, and uricosuric drugs.

Ibuprofen

Dosage: 1.2 g/day to 1.8 g/day in divided doses

Preparation: Oral.

Diclofenac

Usually as an intermediate release diclofenac potassium (Cataflam) or slow release diclofenac sodium (Voltaren)

Dosage: 75–150 mg daily in 2–3 divided doses.

Preparation: Oral, rectal, IM

Tenoxica

Dosage: 20 mg daily.

Preparation: Oral, IM, IV

Piroxicam

Dosage: 10–20 mg as single or divided doses.

Preparation: Oral, IM

Selective Cyclooxygenase-2 (Cox2) Inhibitors

These drugs have less gastrointestinal side-effects profile. Cox1 inhibits prostaglandin synthesis in the gut and platelets while Cox2 inhibit prostanoid mediators of pain, inflammation, fever, and ovulation. Other profiles are similar to NSAIDs.

Celecoxib

Dosage: 200–400 mg as single or two divided doses
Preparation: Oral

Etodolac

Dosage: 600 mg as single or two divided doses
Preparation: Oral

Panecoxib

Dosage: 20–40 mg, 6–12 hourly (start 40 mg)
Preparation: IM/IV

Opioids

Morphine

Mechanism: Opioid receptor agonist

Indication: Moderate to severe pain, postoperative analgesia, standard against which all other opioids are measured.

Side effects: Nausea, vomiting, constipation, palpitation, hypotension, respiratory depression, drowsiness, difficult micturation, allergy, dependence, miosis.

Contraindication: Paralytic ileus, raised intracranial pressure or head injury, respiratory depression, acute alcoholism, pheochromocytoma, ureteric, and biliary colic.

Interaction: Alcohol, amitriptyline, chlorpromazine clomipramine, benzodiazepines, fluphenazine, haloperidol, metochlopramide ritonavir, cimetidine, ciprofloxacin, MAOIs.

Dosage: Acute pain, by IM or SC injection 10 mg 4 hourly if necessary. Chronic pain, oral or SC 5–20 mg every 4 hours

(*oral dose*: IV dose conversion 2:1 to 3:1)

Other routes: IV, rectal.

Dihydrocodeine (DITC)

Mechanism: Weak opioid receptor agonist
Dosage: 30–60 mg every 4–6 hours.

Tramadol

Mechanism: Weak opioid agonist, serotonin, and noradrenaline re-uptake inhibitor.

Comparative side effects: Causes less sedation, constipation, nausea respiratory depression, and less potential for abuse as with other opioids.

Dosage: 50 –100 mg, 6 hourly.

Preparation: IM, IV, oral

Pentazocine

Mechanism: Mixed opioid agonist/antagonist

Indication: Moderate to severe pain

Distinctive side effects: Atrial and pulmonary hypertension, increased myocardial workload. Other side effects include nausea, vomiting, constipation, palpitation, hypotension, respiratory depression, drowsiness, difficult micturition, allergy, dependence, miosis.

Dosage: 30–60 mg, 6 hourly

Preparation: oral, IV, IM, rectal

Pethidine

Mechanism: Powerful opioid agonist, but less potent then morphine

Side effects: Metabolized to nor-pethidine that accumulates in renal dysfunction causing coma and convulsions. Other side effects are similar to those of morphine.

Dosage: 50–100 mg IM, IV or SC 2–3 hourly

Preparation: IV, IM, SC, oral.

Local Anesthetics

Mechanism: Block sodium channels reversibly

Indications: Topical infiltration, wound irrigation, nerve block, epidural and intrathecal blocks.

Side effects: Inebriation feeling, sedation, circum oral paresthesia, twitching, hypersensitivity, convulsions and cardiovascular collapse.

Contraindication/Precaution: IV injection, injection into inflamed tissues, traumatized urethra, in combination with adrenaline in appendages, heart block, hypovolemia.

Lignocaine (Lidocaine, xylocaine)

Onset: 5–10 minutes

Duration: 30–150 minutes

Dosage: Maximum 4 mg/kg plain, 7 mg/kg with adrenaline.

Preparation: Injection, plain and with adrenaline, gel, ointment, heavy (5% in glucose).

Prilocaine

Safe for IV regional block

Dosage: Maximum 400 mg

Distinctive side effects: Methemoglobinemia and cyanosis (treatment: 1% methylene blue at 1 mg/kg IV)

Preparation: Injection

Bupivacaine

Onset: 15–20 minutes

Duration: 4 hours

Dosage: 2 mg/kg/4 hours maximum

Distinctive side effects: Myocardial depression, ventricular fibrillation.

Distinctive contraindication: Biers block

Preparations: Injection with and without adrenaline for nerve blocks, infusion (for Continuous epidural infusion), heavy (0.5% in glucose).

Adjuvants

Adjuvants or "coanalgesics" are employed in the management of neuropathic, visceral, and bone pain. Examples of drugs used as adjuvants in the treatment of pain are as follows.

Tricyclic antidepressants

Amitriptyline

Dosage: 10–25 mg 8 hourly

Gabapentin

Dosage: 100–300 mg daily

Corticosteroids

Biphosphonate

Octereotide
Finasteride, dutasteride
Spasmolytic drugs e.g.1 adrenergic antagonist, antimuscarinic agents (e.g. Oxybutinin hydrochloride).
Nitrite
Pentosan Polysulfate

REFERENCES

1. Merskey H. Pain terms: a list with definitions and notes on usage. Recommended by the IASP subcommittee on Taxonomy. Pain. 1979;6:249–52.
2. Pasero C, Paice JA, McCathery M. Basic mechanism underlying the cause and effects of pain. In: Mathery M, Pasero C Ed. Pain: clinical manual, 2nd ed. St Louis, MO: Moseby;1999:15–34.
3. Cancer pain relief: with a guide to opioid availability, 2nd edn. Geneva. WHO; 1996.
4. Singh A, Alter HJ, Littlepage A. A systematic review of medical literature to facilitate passage of ureteric stones. Ann Emerg Med. 2007;50:552–63.
5. Hwang P, Auclair B, Beechinor D, Dement M, Einarson TR. Efficacy of pentason polysulfate in the treatment of interstitial cystitis: a meta-analysis. Urology. 1997;50:39–43.
6. British National Formulary. BMJ and RPS, London, England. 2008;56:227–50.
7. Burke A, Smyth EM, Fitzgerald GA. Analgesic-antipyretic agents; pharmacology of gout. In: Brunton LL, Lazo JS, Parker KL (Eds). Goodman and Gilman: The pharmacological basis of therapeutics, 11th edn., New York, NY: McGraw-Hill; 2006:671–716.

CHAPTER 2

Antimicrobial Therapy

Ismaila A Mungadi, Hamidu M Liman, Aliu Abdulhameed

■ INTRODUCTION

An understanding of principles and practice of microbial therapy is essential in urology. This is because prompt, adequate, and appropriate therapy using the highly active current drugs has the potential of greatly reducing morbidity and mortality from urologic infections. Appropriate antimicrobial prophylaxis has also reduced infective complications from various endourologic and open procedures.

Urinary tract infection (UTI) is the inflammatory response of urothelium to bacterial invasion. This is said to be simple (or uncomplicated) if it occurs in a healthy patient without anatomic or functional abnormality in the urinary tract, as against complicated infection in which these abnormalities exist.

Antimicrobial therapy may be curative, suppressive, or prophylactic. Cure may not be achieved in a patient with focus of infection or abnormalities that are not resolved.

■ GENERAL PRINCIPLES AND GUIDELINES TO THERAPY

1. Proper assessment and diagnosis must be made, strict criteria should be adhered to in children (Table 2.1).[1]
2. Sensitivity of the uropathogen in question should be evaluated wherever possible. The common uropathogens and their sensitivity pattern should be known in any given environment. This should guide initiation of therapy pending outcome of sensitivity.
3. The pharmacokinetic properties of a given drug, achievable urinary concentration, the drug elimination, half-life, and bioavailability on oral administration should be considered.
4. Potential impediment to bacterial eradication and patient factors permitting bacterial persistence or recurrence such as stone disease, resistance from previous microbial therapy, multi-drug resistant nosocomial pathogens, or possibility of reinfection from vagina, urethra, rectum, or catheters should

Benign Urological Diseases

Table 2.1: Culture criteria for diagnosis of urinary tract infection

Method of Collection	Colony Count (Pure Culture)	Probability of Infection %
Suprapubic Aspiration	Gram-negative bacilli: Any number Gram-positive cocci: More than a few thousand	> 99%w
Catheterization	>10^5 10^4–10^5 10^3–10^4 <10^3	95% Infection likely Suspicious, repeat Infection unlikely.
Clean Catch Voided (Male)	>10^4	Infection likely
Clean Catch Voided (Female)	3 specimens: >10^5 2 specimens: >10^5 1 specimen: >10^5 5 × 10^4–10^5 10^4–5 × 10^4 10^4–5 × 10^4 < 10^4	95% 90% 80% Suspicious, repeat culture Symptomatic; Suspicious; repeat. Asymptomatic; Infection unlikely Infection unlikely

Source: Hellerstein S. Recurrent urinary tract infections in children. Pediatr Infect Dis. 1982;1:271–281.

be considered. The possibilities of fastidious organism such as anaerobes, chlamydia, and mycobacteria should also be considered.
5. Cheaper affordable drugs should be preferred. The course of treatment is more likely to be completed with affordable regimen especially in resource poor settings.
6. The easier and more acceptable the dosage the better the patients' compliance (i.e. oral, once or twice daily dosage).
7 The toxicity of the drug and their effects on the kidney should constantly be kept in mind.

■ ACUTE PYELONEPHRITIS

Escherichia coli infection accounts for majority of cases of acute pyelonephritis. Other pathogens are *Klebsiella, Proteus, Enterobacter, Pseudomonas, Serratia, Citrobacter, Streptococcus faecalis, Staphylococcus saprophyticus, Streptococcus species*, and *Staphylococcus epidermidis*.

Oral therapy for uncomplicated infection may be initiated using trimethoprim-sulphamethoxazole (TMP-SMX), but the fluoroquinolones are more effective. For parenteral therapy, the fluoroquinolones or gentamicin in combination with cephalosporin or ampicillin are effective. Amoxicillin-clavulanic acid can be considered in suspected gram-positive infection. The duration of therapy is generally 7–14 days. Failure of treatment heralds complications of acute pyelonephritis. Complicated infections, relapse, and

Antimicrobial Therapy

Table 2.2: The NIH classification of the prostatitis syndrome

Category	Name	Description
I	Acute bacterial prostatitis (ABP)	Acute infection of the prostate gland
II	Chronic bacterial prostatitis (CBP)	Recurrent infection of the prostate
III	Chronic abacterial prostatitis/ chronic pelvic pain syndrome (CPPS)	No demonstrable infection
IIIA	Inflammatory chronic pelvic pain syndrome (CPPS)	White cells in semen, expressed prostatic secretions or postprostatic massage urine
IIIB	Noninflammatory chronic pelvic pain syndrome (CPPS)	No white cells in semen, expressed prostatic secretions or postprostatic massage urine
IV	Asymptomatic inflammatory prostatitis (histological prostatitis)	No subjective symptoms, detected either by prostate biopsy or by the presence of white cells in expressed prostatic secretions or semen during evaluation of other disorders

Source: Krieger JN, Nyberg LJ, Nickel JC. NIH consensus definition and classification of prostatitis, *JAMA*. 1999;282:236–237.

chronicity must be properly investigated and appropriately treated. Polycystic kidney disease, renal calculi, diabetes mellitus, benign prostatic hypertrophy, steroid therapy, HIV infection, and malignancies are frequent causes of recurrent pyelonephritis.

CYSTITIS

The organisms commonly isolated are *E coli*, *S saprophyticus*, and other *Enterobacteriaceae*. Oral TMP-SMX or fluoroquinolones are effective. Amoxicillin-clavulanic acid or cephalosporins should be considered in pregnancy. Empirical treatment of uncomplicated cystitis should be for 3–7 days. Bacterial persistence and recurrent infections must be investigated. Urinary tract stone, stasis, diverticulum, fistula, foreign bodies, altered vaginal lactobacilli due to menopause, coital habits, and bladder dysfunction are important considerations in patients with bacterial persistence or recurrent infections. Prophylaxis in the prevention of recurrent cystitis can be achieved with nightly doses of nitrofurantoin, TMP-SMX, or fluoroquinolones.

BACTERIAL PROSTATITIS

Bacterial prostatitis may be acute (Type I NIH) or chronic (Type II NIH), (Table 2.2).[2] The most common isolates in bacterial prostatitis are *E coli*, *P aeruginosa*, *Klebsiella species*, other gram-negative *Enterobacteriaceae*, and gram-positive *Enterococci*.

Antimicrobial therapy is the mainstay of treatment of type I and type II prostatitis. Treatment should achieve high intraprostatic drug concentration to be effective. Most drugs achieve high intraprostatic concentration in the acute but not in chronic phase of the disease.

In acute phase, the aim of initial therapy is to achieve high intraprostatic concentration that is best obtained with initial parenteral drugs such as fluoroquinolones, a broad spectrum cephalosporin (e.g. ceftriazone, cefuroxime, cefataxime), or a combination of gentamicin and ampicillin until apyrexia. Therapy is continued with oral fluoroquinolones for up to 4 weeks. The possibility of prostatic abscess should be considered with failure of initial drug treatment.

Drug treatment of chronic bacterial prostatitis is not standardized. Traditional treatment is oral TMP-SMX for up to 13 weeks. Response must be properly evaluated in 4–6 weeks, before continuing therapy. Fluoroquinolones are more effective for shorter duration. Erythromycin and azithromycin are other alternatives. In addition to antibiotics, symptoms relief in patients with chronic prostatitis may require the use of analgesics, nonsteroidal antiinflammatory drugs (NSAIDs), muscle relaxants, alpha blockers, or 5 alpha reductase inhibitors.

■ EPIDIDYMITIS, EPIDIDYMO-ORCHITIS

Epididymo-orchitis secondary to ascending UTI will be related to the urinary pathogen involved in the UTI. Hematogenous spread of *Streptococcal*, *Staphylococcal* or *Proteus* infection may also be the cause. Other causes of epididymo-orchitic are *Neisseria gonorrhoeae*, *Chlamydia trachomatis*, *Haemophilus influenza*, and *Mycobacterium tuberculosis*.

Treatment is according to the causative agent or its likelihood. Treatment is advised for 2 weeks from the state of apyrexia. Doxycycline is the drug of choice for chlamydial infection.

■ GENITOURINARY TUBERCULOSIS

Tuberculosis (TB) may affect the kidneys, ureters, bladder, prostate, urethra, epididymis, testes, or penis. Rifampicin, isoniazid, pyrazinamide, and ethambutol are the first-line anti-tuberculous agents. General measures in the management of tuberculosis should be adhered to. It is also essential to constantly consult current literature on the treatment of tuberculosis, as this is still evolving.

Isolated genitourinary TB can be drug treated for 4–6 months and treatment for more than 6 months is not necessary. Genitourinary TB is responsive to short courses because isoniazid (INH), rifampicin, pyrazinamide and streptomycin achieve high urine concentrations and attain adequate concentration in kidneys, ureters, bladder, and prostate.[3]

URETHRITIS

Gonococcal Urethritis

This is caused by *Neisseria gonorrhoeae*, a gram-negative diplococcus. It is transmitted during vaginal or oral sex with an infected partner and contacts with secretions from the urethra, cervix, pharynx, or anorectum of infected individual. The incubation period varies from 12 hours to 3 months. It produces purulent urethral discharge but may remain asymptomatic, in which the host remains a carrier and potentially infective. To establish diagnosis, calcium alginate urogenital swab should be taken and plated directly unto modified Thayer-Martin selective agar media. Ceftriazone, ciprofloxacin, ofloxacin, doxycycline, erythromycin, or azithromycin are all effective.

Nongonococcal Urethritis

Nongonococcal urethritis caused by *C trachomatis* is treatable with doxycycline, azithromycin, ofloxacin, or erythromycin. It is an advantage to consider these drugs in gonococcal urethritis, since 30% of gonococcal urethritis is associated with chlamydial infection.[4] It must be remembered that the female sexual partner must also be treated.

SYPHILIS AND OTHER SEXUALLY TRANSMITTED INFECTIONS

Syphilis is caused by *Treponema pallidum*. Primary syphilis presents with a painless penile ulcer referred to as chancre. The treatment is single, 2.4 million units, intramuscular (IM) dose of Benzathine penicillin. Penicillin is very effective. The alternative in patients allergic to penicillin is a 2-week course of erythromycin, tetracycline, or doxycycline.

Other sexually transmitted infections amenable to drug treatment that may present to the urologist are lymphogranuloma venereum, granuloma inguinale, chancroid, and pediculosis pubis. Lymphogranuloma venerum is caused by *C trachomatis* and is amenable to treatment with doxycycline, tetracycline, or erythromycin. Doxycycline is more effective. The treatment of granuloma inguinale, caused by *C granulomatis* is tetracycline, doxycycline, or ciprofloxacin.

Chancroid presents as a painful genital ulcer caused by *Haemophilus ducreyi*. The treatment is less predictable due to acquired resistance. Azithromycin, ciprofloxacin, ceftriazone, or erythromycin are recommended.

Phthirus pubis, the crab louse causing pediculosis pubis responds well to treatment with permethrin cream rinse or benzyl benzoate.

GENITAL HERPES

This is caused by a double-stranded DNA virus, Herpes simplex virus types 1 and 2. The drug of choice is acyclovir, which is commonly available as tablets, injection, or cream/ointment. Oral or intravenous acyclovir is more effective than topical. Patients with frequent recurrence can benefit from prophylactic oral acyclovir (200 mg 2–5 times per day)[5] for 3–4 weeks. Valacyclovir is an alternative agent.[6]

MOLLUSCUM CONTAGIOSUM

Molluscum contagiosum is a ubiquitous infection caused by a DNA of the poxvirus family with a high incidence among patients with HIV infection. It is transmitted by intimate skin-to-skin contact. It appears as small umbilicated papules on the skin within which is a milky white material housing the virus. The papules contain molluscum bodies that are spherical masses of eosinophilic hyalin.

Molluscum contagiosum may resolve spontaneously.[7] It may be treated by curetting, evisceration, cryosurgery, or chemical removal using phenol, cantharidin podophyllotoxin cream, silver nitrate, or trichloroacetic acid.

URINARY SCHISTOSOMIASIS

Urinary schistosomiasis is caused by a trematode, *Schistosoma haematobium*. The adult worm resides in the vesical, pelvic, and mesenteric veins but oviposition mainly occurs in the vesical and pelvic veins and venules. Active urinary schistosomiasis essentially results from the schitosome eggs and the vigorous granulomatous host response to them. Chronic urinary schistosomiasis lead to terminal haematuria or vesical complications of chronic cystitis, ulceration, granulomata, polyposis, fibrosis, contracture, epithelial metaplasia, and dysplasia (Fig. 2.1). Chronic urinary schistosomiasis may also involve the bladder neck, ureter, prostate, and urethra. Active schistosomiasis haematobium infection is diagnosed by finding terminally spined eggs in urinary sediments.

Oral praziquantel is now the drug of choice for the treatment of urinary schistosomiasis. The drug combines effectiveness, broad spectrum of activity, and low toxicity. It is active against all schistosomal species. The recommended dosage is 40 mg per kg 2 times a day for 1 day, which may be repeated after 4–6 weeks.[8]

SCROTAL FILARIASIS

Filariasis constitutes a significant health burden in the tropics. Human lymphatic filariasis is caused by *Wuchereria bancrofti*, *Brugia malayi*, and *Brugia timori*, all of which are transmitted by mosquito. The adult

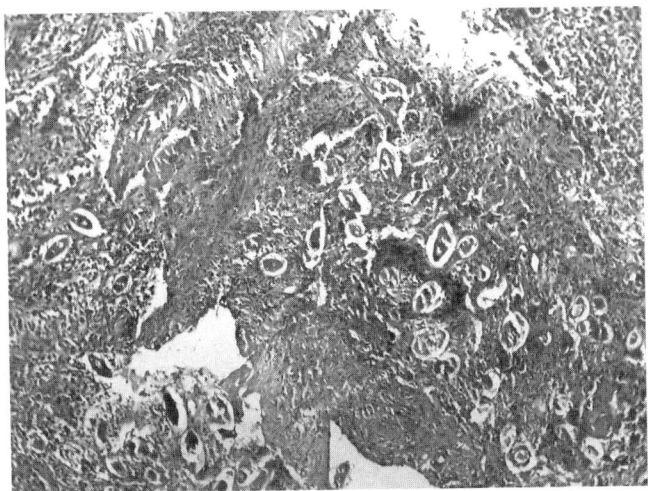

Fig. 2.1: Calcified ova of *Schistosoma haematobium* associated with bladder carcinoma (*For color version, see plate 1*)

Wuchereria bancrofti have predilection for intrascrotal and inguinal lymph vessels where they cause lymphatic inflammation, lymphatic dilatation, and lymphadenopathy leading to lymphatic obstruction and resulting hydrocele and scrotal elephantiasis. The treatment of choice is excision and reconstructive skin cover, as hydroceles and lymphedema will not regress with drugs only.[9]

Medically, control strategies and treatment programs for filariasis have had relative success in disease control and transmission. Drugs have been used singly or in combination. These are Diethyl carbamazine (DEC), ivermectin, and albendazole. DEC is given at 6 mg per kg per day in three divided doses for a period of 2 weeks for both symptomatic and asymptomatic filarial infections. A single oral dose of ivermectin 200–400 μ per kg has a microfilarial clearance comparable to DEC; however, it has no effect on adult filarial, while albendazole eliminates both adult and microfilaria.

FUNGAL INFECTION

Opportunistic

Genitourinary fungal infection is generally on the increase[10] and urologists must be familiar with drug treatment of fungal infections. Candida species are the most common culprits. Patient vulnerability to candida urosepsis is promoted by urinary obstruction, diabetes mellitus, pregnancy, indwelling catheter, antibiotic therapy, invasive monitoring, and immunosuppression. *Candida albicans* is the most frequent isolate. Others are *Candida glabrata* (turulopsis glabrata), *Candida parapsilosis*, *Candida tropicalis*, and *Candida kruzei*.

In immunosuppressed individuals, invasive fungal infection may be caused by Candida species, Cryptococcus species, and Aspergillus species.

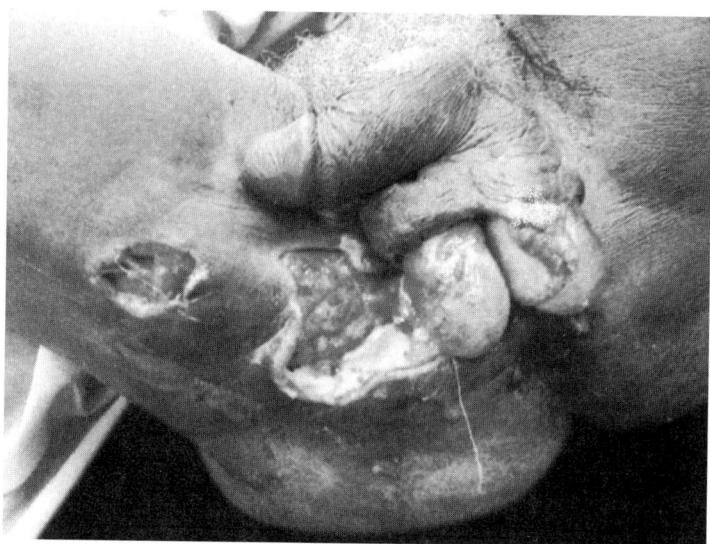

Fig. 2.2: Fournier's gangrene (*For color version, see plate 1*)

A patient with Candida urosepsis may present with systemic candidiasis, cystitis, pyelonephritis, ureteral candida accretion (fungal balls), prostatitis, epididymitis, vulvovaginitis, peristomal infections, or genital skin infections. Active anticandidal agents include nystatin, griseofulvin, fluconazole, ketoconazole, amphotericin B, and various topical imidazole derivatives.

Patients with asymptomatic candiduria may require active therapy and such patients should always be treated before urologic intervention to prevent invasive candidiasis. This can be achieved with oral fluconazole or bladder irrigation with amphotericin B or miconazole.

Tinea infection of the groin, crura, and scrotum is a common tropical infection. The treatment is with topical imidazoles.

ACTINOMYCOSIS

This is caused by a gram-positive anaerobic, rod like, filament forming bacteria that characteristically produce sulfur (yellowish) granules. Actinomycotic infection of the perineum, scrotum, testes, pelvic cavities, bladder, prostate, kidney, and retroperitoneum have been described. The treatment is a long course of penicillins, in initial large doses (please refer to appropriate literature). The alternative drugs are erythromycin and ciprofloxacin.

FOURNIER'S GANGRENE

This is a necrotizing fasciitis of the male genitalia (Fig. 2.2). It is a life-threatening mixed flora infection of the deep cutaneous tissue and fascia. Although infections emanate from the skin, urethra, and rectal areas, predisposing factors such as chronic diseases like diabetes mellitus, perianal sepsis, periurethral infection, circumcision, and trauma have been associated with the disease.

The causative organism is mostly a combination of aerobic and anaerobic bacteria such as *E coli, Klebsiella, Enterococci, Fusobacterium, Bacteroides, Clostridium,* and Streptococcal species. Ulcer base biopsy is characterized by vascular thrombosis, severe necrosis, and subcutaneous tissue necrosis.

Fournier gangrene is a urologic emergency that requires early diagnosis, aggressive treatment with potent antibiotics and surgical debridement to minimize morbidity and mortality. Empirical treatment using ciprofloxacin and clindamycin may be tried. A combination of third-generation cephalosporins such as ceftriaxone and clindamycin may also be used.

■ PERIOPERATIVE ANTIMICROBIAL PROPHYLAXIS

Perioperative antimicrobial prophylaxis is aimed at preventing infection (UTI, wound, and systemic infection) following urologic intervention. There is high incidence of bacteraemia following open or endoscopic procedures in patients with any degree of bacteriuria and this must be treated preoperatively.

Even after eradication of bacteriuria, antibiotic prophylaxis is indicated in the following conditions: transrectal biopsy, urinary obstruction, and when an indwelling catheter or stent is in place. Prophylaxis is also indicated in any procedure utilizing bowel segments, in inplant surgery, during long reconstructive genital operation, and following treatment of infected stones. Immunosuppressed, diabetic, artificial cardiac valves patients, and patients with susceptibility to UTI must be considered for prophylaxis. Prophylaxis should be started at induction of anesthesia or 30–60 minutes before operation for intravenous and 1–2 hours before the start of surgery for oral antibiotics. Though oral fluoroquinolones can be used for prophylaxis, intravenous antibiotics are preferred since they ensure adequate tissue concentration during surgery. A second dose may be necessary if an operation lasts for more than 3 hours. Antibiotic prophylaxis is not necessary for more than 24 hours after surgery.[11]

The antimicrobial selection is based on urologic procedure and the expected micro-organisms in the environment of intervention. There are three potential sources of pathogens:

1. *Urinary tract*: Enterobacteriaceae, Enterococci
2. *Bowel flora*: Enterobacteriaceae, Enterococci, Anaerobes, Streptococci
3. *Wound environment*: Staphylococcus, rarely Streptococci

Therefore, for open and endoscopic procedures on the urinary tract, pathogen in source 1 and 2 should be covered. Fluoroquinolones, cephalosporines, or an aminopenicillin (Ampicillin, Amoxicillin) plus beta-lactam inhibitor (salbactam, clavulanic acid) are all effective.

For urologic operations involving bowel segment or transrectal prostatic biopsy, metronidazole should be added. For operations in which the urinary tract is not opened such as long genital reconstruction and insertion of implants, staphylococci are the main concern. A first-or second-generation cephalosporin or an aminopenicillin plus a β-lactamase inhibitor are effective.

■ OUTLINE OF PHARMACOTHERAPY[12-15]

Aminopenicillins and β-lactamase Inhibitors

Ampicillin/Amoxicillin

Mechanism of action: Bactericidal, inhibit bacterial cell wall synthesis. β-lactam antibiotics.

Activity and indications: Streptococci, sensitive strains of enterobacteriaceae and enterococci. Destroyed by β-lactamase produced by gram-positive and gram-negative bacteria. Addition of β-lactamase inhibitor (e.g ampicillin-salbactam or amoxicillin-clavulanate) extends their spectrum.

Note: Excreted mainly by the kidney (therapeutic concentration in urine), also some hepatic excretion. Dose adjustment is necessary in renal failure.

Side effects: Hypersensitivity, clostridium difficile, pseudomembranous colitis, overgrowth of selected bowel and vaginal flora, and gastrointestinal upset.

Dosage: Amoxicillin: 500 mg to 1 gm every 8 hours, Ampicillin: 500 mg to 1 gm every 8 hours, Sultamicillin: 750 mg twice daily (oral), 1.5 gm to 5 gm every 8 hours (IV), Perioperative prophylaxis 1.5 gm to 5 gm (IV).

Preparation: Ampicillin: Oral, IM, IV; Amoxicillin: Oral, IM, IV; Augmentin (Amoxicillin + clavulanic acid): oral(expressed as Amoxicillin), IV; Sultamicillin (Unasyn, other), (ampicillin + Sulbactam): Oral, IV.

Nitrofurantoin

Mechanism of action: DNA damage. Bacteriostatic at low concentration and bactericidal at high concentration.

Activity and indications: Active against *Escherichia coli* and *Enterococci*. Most species of Proteus and Pseudomonas are resistant. Rapidly excreted in urine to bactericidal concentrations, making it suitable for the prevention and treatment of UTI. These concentrations are not achievable in plasma due to the rapid excretion.

Side effects: Nausea, vomiting, anorexia, diarrhea, pulmonary reaction, hypersensitivity, peripheral neuropathy, hepatitis and cholestatic jaundice, pancreatitis, blood dyscrasia, intracranial hypertension, and transient alopecia.

Contraindications: Infants less than 3 months, impaired renal function, hepatic impairment, G6PD deficiency.

Interaction: Antacids like magnesium trisilicate reduce absorption, uricosuric (e.g. probenacid) reduces excretion. Alkalinization of urine reduces its activity.

Dosage: UTI: 50–100 mg every 6 hours, prophylaxis 50–100 mg at night.

Preparation: Oral.

Cotrimoxazole (Trimethoprim-sulfamethoxazole)

Mechanism of action: Synergistically prevent bacterial tetrahydrofolate synthesis. SMX inhibits incorporation of para-aminobenzoic acid (PABA) into folic acid and TMP inhibits the reduction of dihydrofolate to tetrahydrofolate.

Activity and indications: Activity optimal if administered at ratio 1:5, TMP:SMX. Effective against most uropathogens except *Enterococci* and *Pseudomonas* species. Largely excreted in urine and attain therapeutic levels in vaginal and prostatic secretions. It is effective in acute and chronic UTI, prostatitis, recurrent UTI, and chemoprophylaxis.

Side effects: Nausea, vomiting, exfoliative dermatitis, Steven-Johnson syndrome, toxic epidermal necrolysis, (hypersensitivity reactions common in patients with AIDS) allergic cholestasis, hepatitis, headache, hallucination depression, anemias, and various blood disorders, crystalluria, reversible renal impairment and permanent renal damage in patient with existing renal impairment.

Contraindication: Porphyria, Hypersensitivity.

Precaution: Renal and hepatic impairment, asthma, neonates, pregnancy, breastfeeding predisposition to folate deficiency.

Interactions: Interacts with other sulphonamides and antifolates, methanamine, amiodarone thiopental, prilocaine, warfarin, phenytoin, ciclosporin.

Dosage: 960 mg every 12 hours,

Preparation: Oral, IV.

Fluoroquinolones

Mechanism of action: Potent bactericidal activity by inhibiting bacterial DNA gyrase and topoisomerase IV.

Activity and indications: Fluoroquinolones are active against gram-negative and most gram-positive bacteria, chlamydia and mycobacteria. Activity against streptococci is limited to levofloxacin, gatifloxacin, sparfloxacin, and moxifloxacin and against anaerobe to garenoxacin and gemifloxacin.

Higher than serum levels are achieved in urine, kidneys, prostatic tissue (not secretion). Most are cleared by kidney and dose must be adjusted in renal failure. Levofloxacin, gatifloxacin, lomefloxacin, ofloxacin, ciprofloxacin, fleroxacin have good renal excretion and are suitable for the treatment of UTI.[9] Fluoroquinolones are indicated in the treatment of UTI, prostatitis, gonorrhoeae, chlamydial urethritis, chancroid, and tuberculosis. They are ideal for empirical treatment of UTI.

Side effects: Generally well tolerated, nausea, vomiting abdominal discomfort, colitis, headache, dizziness, hallucination and seizures, orthopathy (children) hypersensitivity, blood disorders, tendonitis, peripheral nervous reactions, and photosensitivity.

Precaution: Epilepsy, myasthenia gravis, pregnancy, children (unless benefits outweigh potential risk of orthopathy), renal damage.

Interaction: NSAID and theophylline increase CNS toxicity; Steroids (increase risk of tendon inflammation), Warfarin (enhanced effects).

Dosage and preparations:

Ciprofloxacin: Oral

UTI: 250–500 mg twice daily.

Chronic prostatitis: 500 mg twice daily

Gonorrhoeae: 500 mg single dose

Preoperative prophylaxis: 750 mg IV infusion (over 30–60 minutes)

UTI: 200–400 mg (400 mg over 60 minutes) twice daily.
Preoperative prophylaxis, 400 mg IV at induction of anesthesia.

Ofloxacin: Oral

UTI: 200–400 mg twice daily.

Chronic prostatitis: 200 mg twice daily for 28 days.

Gonorrhoeae: 400 mg single dose

Nongonococcal urethritis: 400 mg daily for 7 days.
IV infusion (30 minutes per 200 mg)

UTI: 200 mg daily increased to 200–400 mg twice daily in severe infections.

Norfloxacin: Oral

UTI: 400 mg twice daily

Gonorrhoeae: 800 mg single dose.

Perfloxacin: Oral

UTI: 400 mg twice daily

Prostatitis: 400 mg twice daily for 28 days

Gonorrhoeae: 800 mg single dose
Intravenous infusion (over 1 hour) 400 mg.

Cephalosporins

Mechanism of action: Inhibit bacterial cell wall synthesis.

Activity and indications: Cephalosporins are somewhat arbitrarily classified by generation based on antimicrobial activity. **First-generation** cephalosporins such as cephalexin have good activity against gram-positive bacteria (*Streptococci* and *S aureas*) but only modest activity against gram-negative bacteria.

Second-generation drugs such as cefuroxime, have increased activity against gram-negative organisms but not as active against gram-negatives as first generation. The **third-generation** drugs are much more active against *Enterobacteriaceae* and *N gonorrhoeae* and show good activity against gram-positive as well. Ceftazidime is active against *Pseudomonas*. Other third-generation drugs are cefotaxime, ceftriazone and cefpodoxime. The **fourth-generation** cephalosporin (cefepine) has activity similar to third generation and is more resistant to β-lactamases. Excretion of cephalosporins is principally renal.

Side effects: Hypersensitivity, nephrotoxicity, nausea, diarrhea, blood disorders (including thrombocytopenia and platelet dysfunction, leucopenia, and anemia).

Contraindication: Hypersensitivity, porphyria.

Caution: Penicillin sensitivity, renal impairment.

Interaction: Alcohol, antacids, and H_2 antagonist (reduced absorption), anticoagulant, loop diuretic (increased hepatotoxicity), and probenicid (reduced excretion).

Dosage and preparations:

Cephalexin (Ceporex): Oral 500 mg every 8–12 hourly.

Cefuroxime (Zinacef): Oral 250 mg 12 hourly. Gonorrhoeae: 1 gm single dose. IV, IM. 750 mg 3 times daily, Gonorrhoeae: 1.5 gm single dose.

Cefotaxime (Claforan). IV, IM: 1 gm 12 hourly. Gonorrhoea: 1 gm single dose.

Ceftriazone (Rocephin): IV, IM 1 gm daily.

Gonorrhoea: 250 mg single dose.

Perioperative prophylaxis: 1 gm IV. over 2–3 minutes or infusion.

Ceftazidime (Fortum): IM, IV. 1–2 gm every 12 hour.

Preoperative prophylaxis: 1 gm (IM doses of more than 1 gm are divided between more than one site).

Aminoglycoside

Gentamicin

Mechanism of action: Concentration-dependent bactericidal activity by interfering with protein synthesis.

Activity and indications: Active against most gram-negative organism. Not active against anaerobes, *Haemolytic strepococci,* and *Pneumococci.* Gentamicin is useful in complicated UTI and serious gram-negative sepsis. It should be used briefly (not exceeding 7 days) and sparingly due to toxicity. It is usually combined with a penicillin or metronidazole for empirical treatment. Gentamicin should be avoided if organisms are sensitive to other less toxic drugs. Generally, avoid mixing aminoglycosides with other drugs. It is excreted by the kidneys. Periodic determination of plasma concentration is recommended especially in renal impairment and seriously ill patients. The peak concentration is measured from blood sample taken 1 hour after IV. or IM. injection and the trough concentration just before the next dose. A trough concentration persistently above 2 µg per mL is associated with toxicity.[10]

Side effects: The most important side effects of gentamicin are reversible (tubular cells regenerate) nephrotoxicity and irreversible ototoxicity. Reversible nephrotoxicity develops in 8–26% of patient receiving gentamicin for more than several days.[10] The nephrotoxicity is related to the total amount of drug administered and the constancy of elevation above a critical level. Once daily dosing is therefore associated with less nephrotoxicity. Gentamicin produces auditory (cochlear) more than vestibular toxicity. Gentamicin can cause neuromuscular blockade and apnoea.

Contraindications: Myasthenia gravis.

Caution: Renal impairment, pregnancy, infants, elderly, neuromuscular weakness, prolonged use.

Interaction: Increased risk of nephrotoxicity with colistin, vancomycin, amphotericin B ciclosporin, and cisplatin. Increased ototoxicity with vancomycin, neomycin, capreomycin, and cisplatin. Increased risk of neuromuscular blockade with botulinum neurotoxin, nondepolarizing muscle relaxants and antagonizes the effect of neostigmine and pyridostigmine.

Dosage: Multiple dosing: 3–5 mg/kg in three equal doses, 8 hourly IM or slow IV over 3–5 minutes.

Once daily dosing: 5–7 mg/kg IM or slow IV over 30 minutes.

Preparation: IM, IV

Macrolides

Erythromycin, Azithromycin

Mechanism of action: Bacteriostatic. Inhibit protein synthesis by binding reversibly to 50S ribosomal subunits.

Activity and indications: Erythromycin is active against anaerobic gram-positive cocci and bacilli, most strains of *N gonorrhoeae*, *Chlamydia*, and several organisms of no urologic significance. Azithromycin is more active against *N gonorrhoeae* and *Chlamydia* than erythromycin. Macrolide are excreted by the liver (largely) and kidney. Dose adjustment is not necessary in renal dysfunction. Erythromycin and azithromycin are useful alternatives in patients with penicillin allergy. They are also used in urology to treat gonococcal, chlamydial, and actinomycotic (erythromycin) infections. Azithromycin is effective in the treatment of lymphogranuloma venereum.

Side effects: Cholestatic hepatitis and allergy. By acting on motilin receptors, erythromycin stimulates gastrointestinal motility leading to dose-related epigastric discomfort and abdominal cramps. Erythromycin can cause cardiac arrhythmias.

Contraindication: Hypersensitivity, porphyria.

Caution: Hepatic impairment, cardiac arrhythmias.

Interactions: Erythromycin potentiates the effect of carbamazepines, corticosteroids, digoxin, ergot alkaloids, theophylline, and warfarin. Macrolides have potential for very wide interactions that is usually dose related. Manufactures guide should therefore be consulted on this.

Dosage

Erythromycin: Oral 250–500 mg every 6 hours or 500–1000 mg every 12 hours.

Primary syphilis: 500 mg 8 hourly for 14 days.

Chlamydia, nongonococcal urethritis: 500 mg 12 hourly for 14 days.

Lymphogranuloma venereum: 500 mg 6 hourly for 21 days.

Chancroid: 500 mg 6 hourly for 7 days.

Preparation: Oral, IV.

Azithromycin: 500 mg once daily for 3 days.

Lymphogranuloma venereum, granuloma inguinale: 1 gm weekly for 3 weeks
Chlamydial, nongonococcal urethritis 1 gm single dose.

Preparation: Oral.

Metronidazole

Mechanism of action: Electron transfer to metronidazole during anaerobic bacterial metabolism leads to formation of highly reactive nitroradical anions that are bactericidal.

Activity and indication: Active against all anaerobic cocci, anaerobic gram-negative, and anaerobic spore forming gram-positive bacilli. It is also active against a variety of microaerophilic bacteria. Metronidazole is a cheap, versatile drug for the treatment of polymicrobial infections with anaerobic bacteria in urology as well as treatment of *Trichomonas vaginalis* infection and reduction of odor produced by fungating tumors (topical application). Metronidazole is largely eliminated in urine as metabolites with liver as the major site of its metabolism.

Side effects: Nausea, vomiting, metalic taste, headache, dizziness, vertigo, convulsion, allergic reaction, cystitis, dysuria, disulfiram-like effect, hepatitis, jaundice, peripheral neuropathy, blood disorders.

Caution: Carcinogenic in rodents and mutagenic in bacteria, alcohol, hepatic impairment, pregnancy and breastfeeding, prolonged therapy over 10 days.

Interaction: Alcohol, disulfiram, anticoagulants, anti-epileptic, inhibits metabolism of fluorouracil, metabolism inhibited by cimetidine.

Dosage: Oral: 800 mg initially then 400 mg 8 hourly.

Prophylaxis: Oral 400–500 mg 2 hours before surgery.
Rectal 1 gm 2 hourly before surgery.
IV 500 mg at induction.

Preparation: Oral, IV infusion, rectal.

Tetracyclines

Tetracycline

Mechanism of action: Inhibits protein synthesis by binding to 30S bacterial ribosomes. Tetracyclines are bacteriotatic.

Activity and indications: Tetracyclines have a broad spectrum of activity. They are not commonly used for UTI because many UTI-causing bacteria are resistant to tetracyclines. They are, however, encountered in urology for the treatment of lymphogranuloma venereum, various chlamydia-associated infections (nonspecific urethritis, pelvic inflammatory disease, acute epididymo-orchitis), gonorrhoea, granuloma inguinale, syphilis, and actinomycosis. Tetracycline is mainly excreted in the kidney and doxycycline in feces.

Side effects: Nausea, vomiting, diarrhea, pseudomembranous colitis (due to overgrowth of *Clostridium difficile*), photosensitivity, hepatic toxicity, renal toxicity, Fanconi's syndrome (outdated tetracyclines), permanent teeth discoloration (brown) in children, bone growth retardation in infants, blood dyscrasia, benign intracranial hypertension, and hypersensitivity reactions.

Contraindication: Pregnancy, children below 12 years, renal failure (tetracycline).

Caution: Absorption decreased by antacids, aluminum, calcium, iron, magnesium zinc salts, and milk (tetracycline). Other drugs that interact with tetracycline are anticoagulants, anti-epileptics, cyclosporins, ergot alkaloids, estogens, and progesterones.

Dosage: Administer tetracycline 2 hours before or 2 hours after meals or drugs that may interfere with absorption, with plenty of water.

Tetracycline: Generally: 1–2 gm per day in 2–4 divided doses.

Nongonococcal urethritis: 500 mg every 6 hours for 7–15 days.

Syphilis: 500 mg every 6 hours for 14 days.

Preparation: Oral.

Doxycycline

Generally: 200 mg first day then 100 mg 12 hourly.

Primary syphilis: 100 mg twice daily for 14 days.

Nongonococcal urethritis, genital chlamydial infection: 100 mg twice daily for 7–14 days.

Lymphogranuloma venereum: 100 mg twice daily for 21 days.

Preparation: Oral.

Anti-Tuberculous Drugs-First Line

Isoniazid (INH)

Mechanism of action: Isoniazid is a prodrug that is converted into its active metabolite by mycobacterial catalase-peroxidase. It inhibits the synthesis of mycolic acids, which are essential long-branched lipid components of mycobacterial cell wall.

Activity and indication: INH is one of the most effective anti-tuberculous agents.

INH is less effective against atypical mycobacterial organisms. It is bactericidal for actively dividing microorganisms and bacteriostatic for dormant bacilli. It has the ability to penetrate phagocytic cells and is effective against both extracellular and intracellular microorganisms. When given orally or parenterally, adequate plasma concentrations are achieved in 1–2 hours. It diffuses readily into all body fluids and tissues with significant amount in the pleural and ascetic fluids. INH undergoes hydrolysis and acetylation in the liver by *N*-acetyltransferase. It is mainly excreted in urine along with some percentage of the unchanged drug. Individual variation in the metabolism of INH occurs.

Side effects: Hypersensitivity reactions, joint pain, peripheral neuropathy, jaundice, aplastic anemia, optic neuritis, nausea, vomiting, diarrhea, abdominal pain, and constipation

Contraindication: Drug-induced liver disease.

Precaution: Chronic renal failure, diabetes mellitus, hepatic failure, severe malnutrition, and HIV infections. Prophylactic pyridoxine given at 10 mg daily minimizes toxic effects.

Drug interactions: Antacids reduce absorption of INH hepatotoxicity of INH is probably potentiated by general anesthesia and carbamazepine. This drug increases plasma concentration and inhibits metabolism of phenytoin, ethusuximide, diazepam, and theophylline. It reduces plasma concentration of ketoconazole.

Dosage: Oral: 5 mg per kg (4–6 mg/kg) daily maximum of 300 mg daily or 10 mg per kg 3 times weekly (in combination therapy, both adults and children).

IM: injection 200–300 mg per kg single dose (Adult), 10–20 mg per kg daily (children).

Note: Usually prescribed with pyridoxine 10–20 mg daily for the prevention of Isoniazid neuropathy.

Rifampicin

Mechanism of action: Rifampicin is bactericidal. It inhibits RNA synthesis by forming stable complexes with DNA-dependent RNA polymerase. It binds to the β subunit of this complex and inhibits the initiation of RNA chain formation.

Activity and indication: Both intracellular and extracellular microorganisms are killed by rifampicin. It is readily absorbed and penetrates most tissues and phagocytic cells.

It is metabolized by the liver and excreted mainly into the bile, followed by an enterohepatic circulation that results in deacetylation of the drug, thus retaining its complete antibacterial activity and reducing intestinal absorption. Rifampicin is distributed widely in body fluids and tissues including the central nervous system, kidneys, ureter, and prostate. It has a half-life of about 1.5–5 hours.

Side effects: Nausea, vomiting, rashes harmless red-brown discoloration of body fluids (urine, tears, and sweats). Other toxic effects are headache, drowsiness, anemia, renal failure, jaundice, and rarely, hepatitis.

Contraindication: Jaundice, hypersensitivity reactions. Rifampicin must be discontinued permanently when serious side effects develop.

Precaution: Hepatic and renal impairment (may require dose reduction), breastfeeding

Drug interaction: This drug has a wide range of interactions with other agents.

Rifampicin: Reduces plasma concentration (due to increase metabolism) of ACE inhibitors, clarithromycin, dapsone, chloramphenicol, chlorpropamide, carbamazepine, ketoconazole, antiviral agents, and so on. Antacids reduce absorption of rifampicin.

Dosage: 0.6–12 gm daily.

Preparation: Orally or IV infusion.

Pyrazinamide

Mechanism of action: Pyrazinamide is water-soluble, stable analog of nicotinamide. It inhibits mycolic acid synthesis resulting in cell wall disruption by inhibiting the mycobacterial fatty acid synthase I gene. It exhibits bactericidal activity in vitro at acidic pH of about 5.5. Note that tubercle bacilli thrive better in acidic medium.

Activity and indication: It is active against intracellular microorganisms. Pyrazinamide is readily well distributed in the body following oral administrations, and is adequately absorbed through the gut. It has a half-life of about 9–10 hours.

Toxic effects: Hepatotoxicity with jaundice and hepatomegaly, splenomegaly, nausea, vomiting, anemia, and gout.

Contraindications: Acute gouty arthritis.

Precaution: Hepatic failure, diabetes mellitus. Patient's education on symptoms of toxicity is important.

Drug interaction: Pyrazinamide inhibits the action of probenecid and contraceptive effects of estrogens.

Dosage: Adult and children, 25 mg per kg daily or 35 mg per kg, 3 times weekly.

Preparation: Oral.

Ethambutol

Mechanism of action: Ethambutol exhibits its antimycobacterial action by inhibiting arabinosyl transferases. These enzymes polymerize arabinoglycan, an essential component of the mycobacterial cell wall. The inhibition of synthesis of arabinoglycan results in cell wall disruption with increased susceptibility to other drugs.

Activity and indication: Ethambutol is a synthetic, water-soluble, heat stable compound. Ethambutol is administered orally and is readily absorbed from the gut. Plasma concentrations reach a peak, 2–4 hours after administration and have a half-life of 3–4 hours. About half of the drug is excreted in urine unchanged and some in feces.

Side effects: The most important of these is optic neuritis and a decrease in visual acquity, and red/green color blindness. Others are peripheral neuritis and, rarely, rash.

Contraindications: Severe renal impairment, optic neuritis, and poor vision.

Precautions: Doses should be reduced in renal failure. Pregnancy, care is taken in lactating mothers and patients should report visual disturbances when observed and treatment should be terminated.

Drug interaction: Ethambutol is not to be taken with aluminum containing antacids; aluminum decreases the absorption of ethambutol. The agent should not be with BCG.

Dosage: The dose for adult is 1 mg per kg daily or 30 mg per kg, 3 times weekly, and 15 mg per kg daily in children.

Preparation: Oral.

Streptomycin

Streptomycin is a stable, water-soluble aminoglycosidic aminocyclitol. It contains amino sugars linked to aminocyclitol ring by glycosidic bonds. It is derived from Streptomyces griseous. Its hexose ring is a streptidine, which is not centrally positioned; this differentiates it from other aminoglycosides.

Mechanism of action: The precise mechanism by which streptomycin exhibits its bactericidal activity is not well known. However, it causes irreversible inhibition of protein synthesis by binding to the S12 subunit of the ribosomal proteins. This is achieved by its capacity to induce misreading of mRNA and subsequent incorporation of incorrect amino acids, it also disrupts initiation of complex peptide formation and causes fragmentation of polysomes to nonfunctional monosomes. These are concentration-dependent activities.

Activity and indication: Streptomycin is administered parenterally. It is adequately absorbed from site of IM. injection; however, penetration into body fluids and cells is generally poor due to the polar nature of the drug. They bound to plasma albumin, and the plasma concentration reaches its peak after 30–90 minutes after the dose. The half-life is 2–3 hours and the drug is excreted by the kidney in direct relation to the level of creatinine clearance. It is hardly indicated in the treatment of tuberculosis at present.

Side effects: Hypersensitivity reactions, nausea, vomiting skin rashes nephorotoxicity, anemia, pain, and abscess formation from repeated IM injection.

Contraindication: Streptomycin is contraindicated in pregnancy, hearing disorders, and myasthenia gravis.

Precaution: Drug is used with caution in impaired renal function, in infants and elderly where it may be necessary to reduce doses. May possibly be avoided in children because of its painful injection.

Drug interaction: Aminoglycosides, generally, have a wide interaction with other agents; concomitant use of streptomycin with antifungals, ciclosporin, and diuretics increases the risk of nephrotoxicity and ototoxicy.

Dosage: In children and adult by deep IM. 15 mg per kg daily.

Preparation: Intramuscularly

Antiviral Agents

Acyclovir

Mechanism of action: Inhibits viral DNA synthesis.

Activity and indications: Effective against Herpes simplex virus types 1 and 2 and Varicella-zoster virus. Renal excretion is the major route of acyclovir elimination.

Side effects: Nausea, abdominal pain, diarrhea, rashes, pruritis, photosensitivity, allergy, headache, neurotoxicity, and nephrotoxicity. Intravenous acyclovir may cause crystal nephropathy (which resolves with adequate hydration) and severe local irritation.

Caution: Maintain adequate hydration, renal impairment, pregnancy, breastfeeding.

Dosage: Acyclovir, oral.

Herpes simplex: 200 mg 5 times daily for 28 days.

Acyclovir, IV.

Herpes simplex in immunocompromised or severe genital infection: 5 mg per kg over 6 hours for 5 days.
Acyclovir, topical (cream) apply 5 times daily for 5–10 days.

Preparation: Oral, IV, topical.

Others: Valaciclovir, famciclovir. These are available for oral use and as injections. They are administered for shorter duration but are more expensive.

Parasitic Infections

Praziquantel

Mechanism of action: At therapeutic concentrations praziquantel causes influx of calcium across schistosoma tegument and tegumental damage.

Activities and indications: Active against all *schistosoma* species. It is also effective against *Clonorchis sinensis, Opisthorchis viverrini, Fasciolopsis buski, Paragonimus westermani, Hymenolepsis nana, Diphyllobothrium latum,* and *Taenia solium*. It is usually effective for these *trematodes* and *cestodes* at lower doses than for *schistosoma* and *Echinococcus*. Mass treatment of schistosomiasis in endemic areas, therefore, deworms the targeted group against these infestations. Praziquantel is metabolized in the liver (extensive first-pass metabolism) and metabolites are excreted in the kidney. Paraziquantel should be stored at below 30°C.

Side effects: Dose-related nausea, vomiting, abdominal pain, headache, and drowsiness may be observed. Fever, pruritis, rashes, arthralgia, and myalgia are usually related to the worm burden. Severe neurological and ocular reaction may occur in patients with neurocysticercosis or ocular cysticercosis.

Contraindications: Ocular cysticercosis.

Caution: Areas endemic for cysticercosis (cerebral and ocular reaction), tasks requiring skill and mental alertness, hepatic disease, children below 4 years.

Interactions: Bioavailability reduced by hepatic inducers such as phenobarbitone, carbamazepine, and increased by cimetidine.

Dosage: Paraziquantel 40 mg per kg single dose or 2 times in one day. Repeated in 4–6 weeks in severe infestation.

Preparation: Oral.

Diethylcarbamazine (DEC)

Mechanism of action: Its mechanism of action is uncertain; however, it causes microfilarial death, and prevents new lymphatic damage but has no effect on existing lymphatic damage.

Activities and indication: Treatment and prevention of filarial infections. It is a heat stable, water-soluble and odorless compound. It is rapidly absorbed from the gastrointestinal tract with peak concentration in 1–2 hours following single oral dose. It has a half-life of 2–10 hours and is excreted in urine.

Side effects: Compromises specific immune and inflammatory host response by unknown mechanism. Anorexia, headache, nausea, vomiting, dose-dependent retinopathy, encephalopathy, tachycardia, rashes, and headache.

Precaution: Premedication with glucocorticoids and antihistamine may help to reduce reaction to dead microfilarial worms. Use with caution in patients with impaired renal function.

Dosage: To minimize reactions, it is commenced at a dose of 1 mg per kg in day 1 and gradually increased over the next 3 days to 6 mg per kg in divided doses for 2 weeks.

Ivermectin

Mechanism of action: Ivermectin is a semisynthetic analog of an insecticide avamectin B1a. It acts by immobilizing affected organism via a tonic paralysis of the musculature

Activity and indication: It is used extensively in the treatment and control of filariasis, onchocerciasis, and infestations caused by several nematodes and arthropods. It has a half-life of about 57 hours. Peak plasma levels are achieved in 4–5 hours after oral administration and it is mostly bound to plasma protein. It is excreted in urine and gastrointestinal tract.

Side effects: Itching, swollen tender lymph nodes, rashes, tachycardia, myalgia, headache dizziness, hypotension, arthralgia, diarrhea, prostration, facial, and peripheral edema.

Precaution: Avoid concomitant administration with agents that depress CNS activity.

Contraindicating: It interferes with CNS GABA receptors and should not be used in conditions affecting the blood brain barrier such as meningitis and trypanasomiasis. It should not be used in children under 5 years and in pregnancy.

Interaction: Ivermectin induces liver enzymes and as such significantly interacts with drugs that are extensively metabolized by the liver.

Dosage: For lymphatic filariasis, single dose of 200 mcg per kg (together with 400 mg albendazole). This may be repeated at 6–12 months intervals for 5 years, which is based on estimated fecundity of adult filarial worm.

Benzyl Benzoate

Activity and indication: Parasiticidal against Sarcoptes scarbiei and Phthirus pubis.

Side effects: Skin irritation, burning sensation on genitalia.

Caution: Do not shave pubic hair before application (severe burning on excoriated skin), avoid contact with eye or mucous membrane.

Dosage: Apply and wash 24 hours later with soap and water. Repeat if necessary.

Preparation: Topical.

Permethrin

Activity and indications: Parasiticidal against *Phthirus pubis*, *Pediculus humanis capitis*, and *Sarcoptes scarbiei*.

Side effects: Local irritation, pruritis, rashes, and rarely edema.

Caution: Avoid contact with broken skin and mucous membrane, supervise children.

Dosage: Pediculosis pubis: Apply to all body parts (including pubic region and groin) overnight for 12 hours. Repeat after 7 days to kill residual lice from hatched eggs.

Antifungal Agents

Amphotericin B

Amphotericin B is an amphoteric, rigid, almost water-insoluble heptane microlide antibiotic. It is a derivative of *Streptomyces nodesus*. It is characterized by seven conjugated double bonds and a mycosamine, connected to the main ring by glycosidic bond. Its amphoteric property is derived from the presence of a carboxyl and a primary amino group attached to the main ring and mycosamine respectively.

Mechanism of action: Amphotericin B has a characteristic selective antifungal activity. It alters the permeability of the fungal cell membrane by binding strongly to the important and predominant cell membrane sterol, the ergosterol. Its interaction to this cell wall lipid component results in cell wall disruption with development of pores and channels through which a variety of small cell molecule leakages occur.

Activity and indication Absorption of amphoterin B from the gut is very poor; as such for doses to be effective the IV route is used. It is highly protein bound with a half-life of about 15 days and poorly penetrates body fluids and tissues. It is slowly excreted in urine over several days. Hepatic or renal diseases do not appear to affect its metabolism.

Side effects: Infusion related (immediate) side effects include vomiting, headache, fever, chills and hypotension. The intervention is by slowing infusion rate or decreasing daily dose. Late side effects are renal impairment, arrhythmia, hypokalemia, alteration in liver function and hypersensitivity reactions.

Precaution: The toxicity of this drug is concentration dependent; as such, patients should be closely monitored when it is given parenterally. To be used with caution in lactating and pregnant mothers. Monitor hepatic and renal function and avoid rapid IV infusion owing to risk of arrhythmias.

Drug interactions: There is increased risk of nephrotoxicity when used concomitantly with aminoglycosides, ciclosporin, while risk of hypokalemia is more when combined with corticosteroids, cardiac glycosides, loop, and thiazide diuretic.

Dosage: In children and adults, initial test dose of 1 mg over a period of 20–30 minutes is required, followed by 250 μg per kg daily—*see manufactures' guide*.

Preparation: Orally and intravenously.

Imidazoles

Ketoconazole

Ketoconazole is an antifungal imidazole derivative and was the first oral drug used in clinical practice.

Mechanism of action: Ketoconazole inhibits the microsomal cytochrome P450 enzyme. This enzyme is important in the biosynthesis of ergosterol; an essential cytoplasmic component. The resultant effect of its inhibition leads to disruption of membrane bound enzyme systems such as the electron transport system and ATPase enzyme, thus impairing function and growth of the fungi.

Action and indication: It is administered orally. It is metabolized and excreted in the liver and has a half-life of 7–10 hours.

Side effects: Its clinical use is limited by drug interaction and endocrine side effects of gynecomastia, menstrual irregularities, infertility, nausea, and vomiting.

Contraindication: Lactation, severe liver disease, and in hypersensitivity status.

Precaution: Patient should be counseled on symptoms of toxicity in order for him or her to seek immediate medical attention. The drug should be used with care in pregnancy; conditions predisposing to adrenocorticoid deficiency; and avoided in porphyria, renal, and active liver disease.

Drug interactions: It has a wide range of interactions with other agents. An important aspect is effect on drugs metabolized by the liver. Cimetidine appears to inhibit its absorption from the gut.

Dosage: Usually 200 mg daily.

Preparation: Oral
Also, See use in adrenal suppression in cancer of the prostate (Chapter 10).

Miconazole

Miconazole is a synthetic derivative of imidazole. It is mainly used topically against mucosal candidiasis.

Mechanism of action: Its antifungal activity results from inhibition of nucleic acid synthesis and increasing fungal cell membrane permeability to osmotic pressure.

Action indication: Mucosa mycoses

Side effects: Diarrhea, nausea, vomiting, dry mouth, mouth discomfort, upper abdominal pain and gastroenteritis. Others are anemia, leucopenia, thrombocytosis, thrombocytopenia and elevated gamma glutamyltransferase.

Contraindication: Hepatic disorders

Drug interaction: Miconazole increases bleeding tendency in concomitant use with warfarin and may increase side effects of ergot alkaloids, phenytoin and hypoglycemic agents.

Precaution: It should be used with caution in lactating and pregnant mothers.

Dosage: Localized application involves smearing the drug on the affected areas with a clean finger.

Preparation: It is available as sprays, creams, ointment, solution, and powder.

Fluconazole

Fluconazole is a water-soluble fluorinated triazole. It has the widest therapeutic index among the azoles because it has the least effect on hepatic microsomal enzymes.

Mechanism of action: Fluconazole inhibits fungal microsomal cytochrome P450 enzyme called 14 alpha sterol demethylase. This causes impairment in the biosynthesis of ergosterol, an important component of the fungal cell membrane. This results in cell membrane disruption, defects in the close packaging of the acyl chains of the membrane phospholipids and loss of function of certain membrane-bound enzyme systems such as the ATPase and enzymes of electron transport system.

Activity and indication: Fluconazole is administered orally and parenterally. It has an excellent bioavailability by the oral route and a good CSF penetration owing to its water solubility. It is almost completely absorbed from the gut. The drug has a half-life of 22–31 hours and plasma concentration reaches speak of 4–8 µg per mL following successive doses of 100 mg. About 90% of the drug is excreted by the kidney.

Side effects: These include nausea, vomiting, diarrhea, abdominal pain, hepatic disorders, seizures, alopecia, pruritus, and rash. Toxic epidermal necrolysis, erythema multiforme, and hypokalemia.

Precaution: Fluconazole should be used with care in patients with renal impairment or concomitant use with hepatotoxic drugs.

Drug interactions: Fluconazole has a wide range of drug interactions. Concomitant use of fluconazole with other agents increases the side effects of these agents. Fluconazole increases hypoglycemic effect of antidiabetics, and plasma concentration of carbamazepine phenytion, nevirapin, and ritonavir.

Dosage:
Candidal balanitis and vulvovaginal candidiasis: 150 mg single dose
Others—*see manufactures' guide.*

Preparation: Oral (50 mg capsules).

■ REFERENCES

1. Hellerstein S. Recurrent urinary tract infections in children. Pediatr Infect Dis. 1982;1:271–81.
2. Krieger JN, Nyberg LJ, Nickel JC. NIH concensus definition and classification of prostatitis, JAMA. 1999;282:236–7.
3. Johnson WD, Johnson CW, Lowe FC. Tuberculosis and parasitic diseases of the genitor urinary system. In Walsh PC (Ed.), Campbell's Urology, 8th ed., Philadelphia, PA: Sounders; 2002:742–828.
4. Workowski KA, the 1998 CDC. Sexually transmitted diseases treatment guidelines. Curr Infect Dis Resp. 2000;2:44.
5. Douglas JM, Critchlow C, Beneditti J et al. A double-blind study of oral acyclovir for suppression of recurrence at Herpes simplex virus infection. N Eng J Med. 1984;310:1551.
6. Vigil KJ, Chemaly RF. Valacyclovir: approved and off-label uses for the treatment of herpes virus infections in immunocompetent and immunocompromised adults. Expert Opin Pharmacother. 2010;11:1901–13.
7. Cohen J, Powderly WG. Infectious diseases, 2nd ed. New York, NY: Elsevier; 2004:2053–6.
8. The Medical Letter. Drugs for parasitic infections. March 2000.
9. Bernhard P, Magnussen P, Lemnge MM. A randomized, double-blind, placebo-controlled study with diethylcarbamazine for the treatment of hydrocoele in an area of Tanzania endemic for lymphatic filariasis. Trans R Soc Trop Med Hyg. 2001;95:534–6.
10. Wise GJ, Selver DA, Fungal infections of the genitourinary tract J Urol. 1993;149:1377–88.
11. Naber KG, Hofstetter AG, Brühl P, et al. Guidelines for perioperative prophylaxis in urologic interventions of the urinary and male genital tract. Int J Antimicrob Agents. 2001;17:321–6.
12. Naber KG. Which fluroquinolones are suitable for the treatment of urinary tract infection? Int J Antimicrob Agents. 2001;17(4):331–41.
13. Raveh D, Kopyt M, Hite Y, et al. Risk factors for nephrotoxicity in elderly patients receiving once daily aminoglycosides QJ med. 2002;95:291–7.
14. British National Formulary. BMJ and RPS, 2008;56:227–50.
15. Brunton LL, Lazo JS, Parker KL (Eds). Goodman and Gilman's The pharmacological basis of therapeutics, 11th edn., New York, NY: McGraw-Hill; 2006:671–716.

CHAPTER

3

Medical Management of Erectile Dysfunction

Samy Heshmat, Ehab Eltahawy

■ INTRODUCTION

The inability of a male to attain and maintain an erection sufficient to allow sexual intercourse is called erectile dysfunction (ED). It is a part of the general male sexual dysfunction called impotence, which also includes libidinal, orgasmic, and ejaculatory dysfunction.

Only in the past 30 years have we been able to unlock the mysteries of the functional anatomy and the pathophysiology of erection, and consequently understand erectile dysfunction. In addition to the role of smooth muscle in regulating arterial and venous flow, the three-dimensional structure of the tunica albuginea and its role in venous occlusion were elucidated. Also the identification of nitric oxide (NO) as the major neurotransmitter for erection and of phosphodiesterases (PDEs) for detumescence, has had major impact on how we treat this disease.

■ PATIENT EVALUATION

The first step in evaluating ED is always a detailed medical and psychological history of patients and partners.[1]

Medical History

The goals of medical history-taking are to evaluate the potential role of underlying medical conditions (e.g. atherosclerosis, diabetes) and comorbidities (e.g. depression); to differentiate between potential organic and psychogenic causes; and to assess the potential role of medication.

Sexual History

This may include information about previous and current sexual relationships, current emotional status, onset and duration of the erectile problem, and previous consultations and treatments. A detailed description should be made of the rigidity and duration of both erotic and morning erections.

The complete International Index of Erectile Function (IIEF) is a questionnaire composed of 15 questions; an abridged 5-item version, called the sexual health inventory for men (SHIM), has been developed and validated, they help objectively evaluate sexual function as well as the impact of a specific treatment modality.[2]

Psychosocial History

A detailed psychosocial assessment is essential. Given the interpersonal context of sexual problems, the physician should carefully assess the patient's past and present partner relationships.

Social history also provides valuable information. Life stressors such as change in social status, divorce, death of spouse, loss of job, or family problems may have an effect on erectile function.

Physical Examination

It should include a general screening for medical risk factors or comorbidities, such as body habitus (secondary sexual characteristics), and an assessment of the cardiovascular, neurologic, and genital systems.

Evaluation of sexual and genital development may occasionally reveal an obvious cause (e.g., micropenis, chordee, Peyronie's plaque).

Laboratory Testing

Laboratory testing must be tailored to the patient's complaints and risk factors. All patients must undergo a fasting glucose and lipid profile if not assessed in the previous 12 months. Hormonal tests must include a morning sample of total testosterone level.

Additional hormonal tests, for example prolactin, follicle-stimulating hormone (FSH), luteinizing hormone (LH), must be carried out when low testosterone levels are detected.

Specialized Diagnostic Tests

Most patients with ED can be managed within the sexual care setting, but some patients may need specific diagnostic tests: Patients with primary erectile disorder; young patients with a history of pelvic or perineal trauma; patients with penile deformities that might require surgical correction; patients with complex psychiatric or psychosexual disorders; patients with complex endocrine disorders

Nocturnal penile tumescence and rigidity: Should only be performed in younger males, that is less than 60 years of age, in which the etiology of the impotence is not obvious and in all patients, no matter what their age, if there is a need to differentiate psychological from organic causes for the sexual dysfunction.

The nocturnal penile tumescence and rigidity (NPTR) assessment should be done on at least two nights. A functional erectile mechanism is indicated by an erectile event of at least 60% rigidity recorded on the tip of the penis that lasts for 10 minutes or more.[3] Patients with a psychological cause for their impotence will have normal sleep erection cycles, whereas patients who have a physical cause (organic) will have some abnormality of the frequency, intensity, or duration of their sleep erections.

Duplex ultrasound of penile arteries: Radiological imaging in the field of erectile dysfunction has diminished in importance over the past 5 years with the advent of new therapies. However, in selected cases, Doppler scanning continues to have a role, and current research is aimed at optimizing the results of the tests. Doppler assessment is performed after intracavernosal injection of a vasoactive pharmacologic agent to induce and maintain an erection. A peak systolic blood flow higher than 30 cm per second and a resistance index higher than 0.8 are generally considered normal.[4] Further vascular investigation is unnecessary when a Duplex examination is normal.

Arteriography and Dynamic Infusion Cavernosometry or Cavernosography

Arteriography and dynamic infusion cavernosometry or cavernosography (DICC) should be performed only in patients who are being considered for vascular reconstructive surgery.[5]

Neurological Studies

Currently, there is no reliable clinical test of the neurologic function of the corpus cavernosum. Neurologic tests of dorsal penile nerve function and sensory function of the genitalia can be performed, but these tests do not assess directly the neurologic function of the corpus cavernosum and do not replace specialized neurourological evaluation by a neurologist.[6]

■ TREATMENT OF ERECTILE DYSFUNCTION

The chosen treatment should meet the needs, preferences, and expectations of the patient and his partner. The primary goal is to determine the etiology of the disease and treat it when possible, and not to treat the symptom alone.

As a rule, ED can be treated successfully with current treatment options, but cannot be cured. The only exceptions are psychogenic ED, posttraumatic arteriogenic ED in young patients and hormonal causes, which can be potentially cured with specific treatment.

Most men with ED will be treated with treatment options that are not cause specific. This results in a structured treatment strategy that depends on efficacy, safety, invasiveness, and cost, as well as patient preference.[7]

Both specific and nonspecific treatments are now available. The former includes lifestyle change, psychosexual therapy, replacement of offending medications, and hormonal therapy; the latter includes oral phosphodiesterase type-5 (PDE-5) inhibitors, intracavernous injection, intraurethral applications, and the vacuum constriction device.

Lifestyle Change

Lifestyle changes and risk factor modification must precede or accompany ED treatment. Some studies have suggested that the therapeutic effects of PDE-5 inhibitors may be enhanced when other comorbidities or risk factors are aggressively managed.[8]

Medication Change

Changing the medications that are well known to cause ED is a reasonable first step in treatment. In many situations, changing to a different class of medication is a feasible first step. For example, nonspecific α-adrenergic blockers clinically have the most severe effects on erectile function. Also, SSRIs are known to cause treatment-related arousal disorders in as high as 70% of patients.[9]

Psychosexual Therapy

Both partners should be willing to participate and cooperate with therapy. Major relationship problems should be addressed before therapy is introduced. Similarly, major stresses with work, finances, or family will need to be evaluated and corrected first.

More recent approaches to sex therapy have included cognitive-behavioral interventions focused on challenging or correcting maladaptive cognitions, behavioral techniques and psychodynamic explorations exploring the role of past developmental experiences on present behavior, and systemic and couples therapy.

Vacuum Constriction Device

The least invasive ED treatment options, apart from psychosexual counseling, are vacuum erection (constriction) devices. Vacuum devices consist of an external cylinder fitted over the penis, which pumps out air and allows the penis to fill with blood; a constriction ring around the base of the penis maintains the erection. To avoid injury, the ring should not be left in place for longer than 30 minutes. The devices are particularly useful in patients who need help initiating and maintaining an erection, such as patients who have undergone radical prostatectomy or have veno-occlusive dysfunction. Vacuum devices are also appropriate following penile vascular surgery or in men with a malfunctioning penile prosthesis in place, and after explantation to prevent shortening.[10] In men with severe vascular insufficiency, combining intracavernous injection with the vacuum constriction device may enhance the erection.[11]

Relative contraindications include severe penile deformity; sickle-cell disease; bleeding disorder or anticoagulation therapy. The commonest adverse events include pain, inability to ejaculate, petechiae, bruising, and numbness, which occur in less than 30% of patients.[12]

Hormonal Therapy

Testosterone replacement therapy (intramuscular, oral, or transdermal) is effective in patients with hypogonadism, but should only be used after other endocrinological causes for testicular failure have been excluded; Hypogonadism is the clinical syndrome with characteristic symptoms and signs associated with low testosterone usually a morning sample, with free testosterone measurement. Symptoms include decreased libido, erectile dysfunction, decreased spontaneous erections. Non sexual symptoms include reduced energy, depressed mood, and increased body fat. A trial of therapy for 3-6 months is reasonable with goal being symptomatic improvement then reassess. Injectables (testosterone cypionate/enanthate q1-3 weaks) has the disadvantage of level fluctuations. Testesterone pellet implants require surgical procedure and lasts 3 months. Topical gels can have variable absorption and patient should be aware of transfer to partner. Oral forms have short half life and significant liver toxicity.

Recent reports suggest a marginal synergistic effect when testosterone is added to PDE-5 inhibitors in hypogonadal men in whom the latter failed as a single therapy.[13] It is contraindicated in men with a history of prostate carcinoma. The hematocrit level should be monitored, as it causes significant erthrocystosis, and a dose adjustment of testosterone may be necessary, especially in congestive heart failure.

OUTLINE OF PHARMACOLOGIC THERAPY

Peripherally Acting Agents

Oral Therapy

Oral agents are considered to be the first-line treatment for patients with ED.

Phosphodiesterase type-5 inhibitors: The normal pathway for penile erection is initiated by sexual arousal, which stimulates release of NO at nerve endings in the penis and from vascular endothelial cells. NO diffuses into vascular and cavernous smooth muscle cells in the corpus cavernosum to cause stimulation of guanylyl cyclase and elevation of cyclic guanosine monophosphate (GMP)

Table 3.1 Common adverse events of the three PDE-5 inhibitors used to treat ED

Adverse Event	Sildenafil	Tadalafil	Vardenafil
Headache	12.8%	14.5%	16%
Flushing	10.4%	4.1%	12%
Dyspepsia	4.6%	12.3%	4%
Nasal congestion	1.1%	4.3%	10%
Dizziness	1.2%	2.3%	2%
Abnormal vision	1.9%		< 2%
Back pain		6.5%	
Myalgia		5.7%	

*Adapted from EMEA statements on product characteristics.

in these cells. This leads to hyperpolarization and lowering of cytoplasmic calcium, which in turn results in smooth muscle relaxation with resultant increased blood flow and penile erection.

The PDE-5 enzyme hydrolyzes cyclic guanosine monophosphate (cGMP) in the cavernosum tissue of the penis. Inhibition of PDE-5 results in potentiation of the effect of the NO. Without sexual stimulation and resultant NO release, these inhibitors are ineffective.[14]

The currently available PDE-5 inhibitors include Sildenafil, Tadalafil, and Vardenafil. Despite the lack of direct comparative studies, all three PDE-5 inhibitors appear to have equivalent efficacy in the treatment of ED. All appear to be generally well tolerated and have similar contraindications and warnings (Table 3.1).

Sildenafil: Sildenafil is effective from 30 to 60 minutes after administration. It is administered in 25, 50, and 100 mg doses. The recommended starting dose is 50 mg and should be adjusted according to the patient's response and side effects. It is effective for up to 12 hours.[15] The efficacy of sildenafil in almost every subgroup of patients with ED has been successfully established.

Tadalafil: Is effective from 30 minutes after administration, with peak efficacy after about 2 hours. Efficacy is maintained for up to 36 hours.[16] It is administered in 10 and 20 mg doses. The recommended starting dose is 10 mg and should be adjusted according to the patient's response and side effects. Tadalafil also improved erections in difficult-to-treat subgroups. Tadalafil, 5 mg once daily, was shown to be well tolerated and effective.[17] This provides an alternative to on-demand dosing of tadalafil for couples who prefer spontaneous rather than scheduled sexual activities.

Vardenafil: Is effective from 30 minutes after administration. It is administered in 5, 10, and 20 mg doses. The recommended starting dose is 10 mg and should be adjusted according to the patient's response and side effects. In vitro, it is 10-fold more potent than sildenafil, though this does not necessarily mean greater clinical efficacy.[18]

Safety Issues for PDE-5 Inhibitors

Cardiovascular safety: Patients who seek treatment for sexual dysfunction have a high prevalence of cardiovascular disease. This places them at risk for adverse events during sexual activity due to the physiologic stress posed on the heart. Those patients can be stratified into three cardiovascular risk categories, which can be used as the basis for initiating or resuming sexual activity.

Low-risk category: The low-risk category includes patients who do not have any significant cardiac risk associated with sexual activity. Low risk is typically implied by the ability to perform exercise of modest intensity. They do not need cardiac testing or evaluation before the initiation or resumption of sexual activity or therapy for sexual dysfunction.

Intermediate-risk category: The intermediate- or indeterminate-risk category consists of patients with an uncertain cardiac condition or patients whose risk profile requires testing or evaluation before the resumption of sexual activity.

High-risk category: High-risk patients have a cardiac condition that is sufficiently severe and/or unstable for sexual activity to carry a significant risk. Sexual activity should be stopped until the patient's cardiac condition has been stabilized by treatment or a decision made by the cardiologist and/or internist that it is safe to resume sexual activity.

Nitrates are totally contraindicated with PDE-5 inhibitors: Organic nitrates and other nitrate preparations used to treat angina, are absolute contraindications with the use of PDE-5 inhibitors. They result in cGMP accumulation and unpredictable falls in blood pressure.

Antihypertensive drugs: Co-administration of PDE-5 inhibitors with antihypertensive agents may result in small additive drops in blood pressure, which are usually minor.

Alpha-blocker interactions: All PDE-5 inhibitors show some interaction with alpha-blockers, which may result in orthostatic hypotension. Sildenafil 50 or 100 mg should not be taken within 4 h following treatment with an alpha-blocker. Tadalafil is contraindicated in patients taking alpha-blockers, except for tamsulosin, 0.4 mg.[19]

Management of Nonresponders to PDE-5 Inhibitors

The two main reasons why patients fail to respond to a PDE-5 inhibitor are either incorrect drug use or inefficacy of the drug.

The main ways in which a drug may be incorrectly used are as follows:
- Failure to use adequate sexual stimulation
- Failure to use an adequate dose
- Failure to wait an adequate amount of time between taking the medication and attempting sexual intercourse.

Other Oral Agents

Apomorphine sublingual: Apomorphine is a centrally acting dopamine agonist that improves erectile function by enhancing the natural central erectile signals that normally occur during sexual stimulation.[20,21] It is administered sublingually on demand in 2 or 3 mg doses. Apomorphine has been approved for ED treatment in several countries but not in the USA.

Yohimbine: Yohimbine is a centrally and peripherally active alpha-2 adrenergic antagonist used as an aphrodisiac for almost a century.

Delequamine: is a more specific and selective alpha-2 adrenergic antagonist than yohimbine.

Trazodone: Trazodone is a serotonin reuptake inhibitor (antidepressant) associated with prolonged erections and priapism. It is also a non-selective alpha-adrenergic antagonist in the corporal smooth muscle cells.

L-arginine: L-arginine is an NO donor and nalmefene/naltrexone is an opioid-receptor antagonist.

Limaprost: Limaprost is an *alprostadil* derivative for oral use.

An oral formulation of phentolamine (nonselective alpha-adrenergic antagonist) has undergone phase III clinical trials.[22]

Intracavernous Injections (ICI)

Approximately 30% of patients do not respond to PDE-5 inhibitor therapy, and another 15% have contraindications. For these men, ICI or transurethral therapy with vasoactive agents may be indicated.

Papaverine: It is a nonselective inhibitor of PDE, leading to increased cyclic AMP and cyclic GMP in penile erectile tissue. The main advantage is its low cost. The major disadvantages are the incidences of priapism (up to 35%) and corporeal fibrosis (1% to 33%), thought to be a result of low acidity. It is only used in combination therapy today due to its high incidence of side effects as monotherapy.

Phentolamine methylate: It is a nonselective, competitive α-adrenoceptor antagonist. Its main side effects include sytemic hypotension, reflex tachycardia, nasal congestion, and gastrointestinal upset. As monotherapy, it produces a poor erectile response. It is used mainly in combination therapy to increase efficacy.

Alprostadil (Prostaglandin E_1): Refers to the exogenous form of PGE_1. It is the most efficacious monotherapy for intracavernous treatment in 5–40 µg doses. The erection appears after 5–15 minutes and lasts according to the dose injected. Efficacy rates for intracavernous alprostadil are more than 70%.[23] Complications of intracavernous alprostadil include penile pain (50% of patients), prolonged erections (5%), priapism (1%), and fibrosis (2%).[24] Pain is usually self-limited after prolonged use. It can be alleviated with the addition of sodium bicarbonate or local anesthesia.[25,26] Fibrosis requires temporary discontinuation of the injection program for several months. Systemic side effects are uncommon.

Combination therapy: Papaverine (7.5–45 mg) plus phentolamine (0.25–1.5 mg), and papaverine (8–16 mg) plus phentolamine (0.2–0.4 mg) plus alprostadil (10–20 µg), have been widely used with improved efficacy rates.

The triple combination regimen had the highest efficacy rates, reaching 92%; this combination had similar side effects as alprostadil monotherapy, but a lower incidence of penile pain due to lower doses of alprostadil. However, fibrosis was more common (5–10%) when papaverine was used.

Transurethral (TU) Alprostadil

For post-surgical or needle-phobic patients who cannot use or choose not to use oral agents, TU vasoactive treatment may be more suitable. Alprostadil, the synthetic formulation of PGE_1, is the only pharmacologic agent with FDA approval for ED. The medicated urethral system for erection (MUSE; Vivus, Inc, Mountain View, CA) consists of a very small semisolid pellet (3 × 1 mm) administered into the distal urethra (3 cm) by a proprietary applicator (MUSE).

Success rate is in the range of 30–65.9% of patients. Higher doses (500 and 1,000 µg) have to be used to produce an adequate clinical response.[27–29] The application of a constriction ring at the root of the penis may improve efficacy.

The most common adverse events are local pain (29–41%) and dizziness (1.9–14%). Urethral bleeding (5%) and urinary tract infections (0.2%) are adverse events related to the mode of administration.

■ REFERENCES

1. Hatzichristou D, Hatzimouratidis K, Bekas M, et al. Diagnostic steps in the evaluation of patients with erectile dysfunction. J Urol. 2002;168(2):615–20.
2. Rosen RC, Riley A, Wagner G, et al. The international index of erectile function (IIEF): a multidimensional scale for assessment of erectile dysfunction. Urology. 1997; 49(6):822–30.
3. Hatzichristou DG, Hatzimouratidis K, Ioannides E, et al. Nocturnal penile tumescence and rigidity monitoring in young potent volunteers: reproducibility, evaluation criteria and the effect of sexual intercourse. J Urol. 1998;159(6):1921–26.
4. Wespes E, Schulman C. Venous impotence: pathophysiology, diagnosis and treatment. J Urol. 1993;149(5 Pt 2):1238–45.
5. Bemelmans BL, Hendrikx LB, Koldewijn EL, et al. Comparison of biothesiometry and neuro-urophysiological investigations for the clinical evaluation of patients with erectile dysfunction. J Urol. 1995;153(5):1483–86.
6. Hatzichristou D, Rosen RC, Broderick G, et al. Clinical evaluation and management strategy for sexual dysfunction in men and women. J Sex Med. 2004;1(1):49–57.

7. Guay AT, Optimizing response to phosphodiesterase therapy: impact of risk-factor management. J Androl. 2003;24(6 Suppl):S59-S62.
8. Montejo-Gonzalez AL, Llorca G, Izquierdo JA, et al. SSRI-induced sexual dysfunction: fluoxetine, paroxetine, sertraline, and fluvoxamine in a prospective, multicenter, and descriptive clinical study of 344 patients. J Sex Marital Ther. 1997;23(3):176-94.
9. Sundaram CP, Thomas W, Pryor LE, et al. Long-term follow-up of patients receiving injection therapy for erectile dysfunction. Urology. 1997;49(6):932-5.
10. Marmar JL, DeBenedictis TJ, Praiss DE, The use of a vacuum constrictor device to augment a partial erection following an intracavernous injection. J Urol. 1988;140(5):975-9.
11. Lewis RW, Witherington, R. External vacuum therapy for erectile dysfunction: use and results. World J Urol. 1997;15(1):78-82.
12. Greenstein A, Mabjeesh NJ, Sofer M, et al. Does sildenafil combined with testosterone gel improve erectile dysfunction in hypogonadal men in whom testosterone supplement therapy alone failed? J Urol, 2005;173(2):530-2.
13. Shabsigh R. Hypogonadism and erectile dysfunction: the role for testosterone therapy. Int J Impot Res. 2003;15(Suppl 4):S9-S13.
14. Lue TF. Erectile dysfunction. N Engl J Med. 2000;342(24):1802-13.
15. Moncada I, Jara J, Subirá D, et al. Efficacy of sildenafil citrate at 12 hours after dosing: re-exploring the therapeutic window. Eur Urol. 2004;46(3):357-360; discussion 360-1.
16. Porst H, Padma-Nathan H, Giuliano F, et al. Efficacy of tadalafil for the treatment of erectile dysfunction at 24 and 36 hours after dosing: a randomized controlled trial. Urology. 2003;62(1):121-5; discussion 125-6.
17. Porst H, Rajfer J, Casabé A, et al. Long-term safety and efficacy of tadalafil 5 mg dosed once daily in men with erectile dysfunction. J Sex Med. 2008;5(9):2160-69.
18. Bischoff E, Niewoehner U, Haning H, et al. The oral efficacy of vardenafil hydrochloride for inducing penile erection in a conscious rabbit model. J Urol. 2001;165(4):1316-18.
19. Auerbach SM, Gittelman M, Mazzu A, et al. Simultaneous administration of vardenafil and tamsulosin does not induce clinically significant hypotension in patients with benign prostatic hyperplasia. Urology. 2004;64(5):998-1003; discussion 1003-4.
20. Hagemann JH, Berding G, Bergh S, et al., Effects of visual sexual stimuli and apomorphine SL on cerebral activity in men with erectile dysfunction. Eur Urol. 2003;43(4):412-20.
21. Montorsi F, Perani D, Anchisi D, et al. Brain activation patterns during video sexual stimulation following the administration of apomorphine: results of a placebo-controlled study. Eur Urol. 2003;43(4):405-11.
22. Goldstein II, Oral phentolamine: an alpha-1, alpha-2 adrenergic antagonist for the treatment of erectile dysfunction. Int J Impot Res. 2000;12(S1):S75-S80.
23. Linet OI, Ogrinc FG. Efficacy and safety of intracavernosal alprostadil in men with erectile dysfunction. The Alprostadil Study Group. N Engl J Med. 1996;334(14):873-77.

24. Chen RN, Lakin MM, Montague DK, et al. Intracavernous injection therapy: analysis of results and complications. J Urol. 1990;143(6):1138–41.
25. Kattan S. Double-blind randomized crossover study comparing intracorporeal prostaglandin E1 with combination of prostaglandin E1 and lidocaine in the treatment of organic impotence. Urology. 1995;45(6):1032–6.
26. Moriel EZ, Rajfer J. Sodium bicarbonate alleviates penile pain induced by intracavernous injections for erectile dysfunction. J Urol. 1993;149(5 Pt 2): 1299–1300.
27. Guay AT, Perez JB, Velásquez E, et al. Clinical experience with intraurethral alprostadil (MUSE) in the treatment of men with erectile dysfunction. A retrospective study. Medicated urethral system for erection. Eur Urol. 2000;38(6): 671–6.
28. Fulgham PF, Cochran JS, Denman JL, et al. Disappointing initial results with transurethral alprostadil for erectile dysfunction in a urology practice setting. J Urol, 1998;160(6 Pt 1):2041–6.
29. Mulhall JP, Jahoda AE, Ahmed A, et al. Analysis of the consistency of intraurethral prostaglandin E(1) (MUSE) during at-home use. Urology. 2001;58(2): 262–6.

CHAPTER

4

Medical Treatment of Urinary Incontinence

Ayman Mahdy, Ismaila A Mungadi

■ INTRODUCTION

As defined by the International Continence Society, urinary incontinence (UI) is "the complaint of any involuntary leakage of urine."[1] Many types of UI have been defined with the most common being stress urinary incontinence (SUI), urge urinary incontinence (UUI), and mixed urinary incontinence (MUI). SUI is the complaint of involuntary leakage on effort or exertion, or on sneezing or coughing. UUI is the complaint of involuntary leakage accompanied by or immediately preceded by urgency. MUI, however, is the complaint of involuntary leakage associated with urgency and also with exertion, effort, sneezing, or coughing.[1] UI is a major health problem that affects both men and women with higher prevalence in women and among aging populations. UI significantly affects patients' quality of life with possible subsequent stigmatization.[2]

■ CONTROL OF MICTURITION

The parasympathetic (S_2-S_4) efferent is excitatory to the detrusor muscle and passes through the pelvic splanchnic nerves to reach the bladder via the inferior hypogastric plexus. The sympathetic (T_{12}-L_2) efferent passes through hypogastric plexus. The sympathetic nerves stimulate α-adrenergic receptors concentrated in the trigone, bladder neck, and urethra. The striated external sphincter is innervated by pudendal nerves. The afferents pass through similar pathways to the spinal cord. Bladder afferent consists of myelinated (A-δ) and unmyelinated (C) fibers. These afferents monitor bladder tension and volume. Silent C fibers become recruited as mechanoreceptors in response to various chemical stimuli.

Normal continence is promoted by spinal guarding reflex. This is brought during sympathetic stimulation caused by bladder distension during filling. The outlet smooth muscles and urethral sphincter contract while the parasympathetic bladder muscular activity is inhibited. Intense bladder activity activates the pontine micturition center and micturition is initiated by inhibition of this guarding reflex. Micturition can be voluntarily aborted by contracting periurethral sphincter that also reflexly inhibits detrusor contraction.

EVALUATION OF URINARY INCONTINENCE PATIENTS

Starting with the patient history, a thorough evaluation should detect all aspects of the patients' condition. History should identify the type of UI, severity (number of pads, diapers, or other protection methods used per day), impact on quality of life using certain validated questionnaires, age at onset, previous treatment trials, associated medical conditions (especially gastrointestinal, neurological, and/or mental). History might also help identifying certain reversible causes of UI. Associated storage and/or emptying urinary tract symptoms should be addressed.

HOW CAN WE PREVENT URINARY INCONTINENCE?

The first and most important step in treating disease conditions is prevention. Although it seems difficult, prevention of UI has been a potential project for many health organizations including the National Institute of Health (NIH).[3] Proper recognition of the risk factors for the condition is an important step during the prevention process. The risk factors for UI include advanced age, gender (females more than males), diabetes, neurological diseases, pregnancy and childbirth, smoking, obesity, urinary tract infections (UTIs), history of UI during childhood, positive family history of UI, physical inability, use of other medications, pelvic organ prolapse (POP), cognitive diseases, as well as menopause in women and prostate diseases in men. Lifford et al.[4] have summarized the potential target populations for urine incontinence prevention. Those populations included the following:

1. *Pregnant women*: Pelvic floor muscle training (PFMT) during pregnancy and the postpartum period has been shown to decrease the UI rates during late pregnancy and postpartum.
2. *Post-prostatectomy incontinence*: Pre- and postoperative PFMT was shown to decrease the prevalence of SUI in this group of patients.[5]
3. *Elderly population*: Diokno et al.[6] have reported that combined bladder training and PFMT have doubled the continence rate in the studied elderly women 55 to 80 years of age.
4. *Diabetic patients*: Prevention of diabetes mellitus type 2 could prevent almost half of severe incontinence conditions.

URINARY INCONTINENCE MANAGEMENT OPTIONS

Many lines of treatment have been studied in the literature. The approach is usually a combination of different therapies. A list of the medical management options is summarized below:

1. *No treatment*: The "no treatment" approach is considered after underlying medical conditions (tumors, cancer, urinary retention, urinary obstruction etc.) have been excluded. A second important factor that affects the "no treatment" decision is the patient choice.
2. *Conservative management*: This includes bladder retraining, toilet training, timed voiding, PFMT, general advice (fluids, diet, and bowel management), medication review, management of bowel dysfunction (constipation/fecal impaction), improving access to toilet facilities, and improving mobility and use of pads/continence aids and other supplies:
   a. *Bladder retraining*: is considered the first-line treatment for UI.[7] Through this approach, the patient is taught how to suppress the urgency "wave." There are few strategies the patient can follow; these include distraction (thinking of something different from the sensation of urgency), repeated pelvic floor muscle contractions (rapid and intense 5–6 contractions within 2–3 seconds), toe pressure, and perineal pressure (patients may sit on their heel). This increases the scheduled interval between voiding by 30 minutes.
   b. *PFMT* is prescribed as first-line treatment for SUI, UUI. or MUI, particularly in cases with no concomitant POP.[8] It is based on "Kegel" exercise and consists of repetitive contractions of the PFM. It is taught by a health care provider. Midwives can be responsible for postpartum rehabilitation using this technique as well. Voluntary contraction of the PFM helps to increase the urethral pressure, improves SUI, and also suppress detrusor muscle contraction and hence improves UUI.

The first step is to help the patient identify the correct muscles. The patient is asked to act as if he or she is trying to prevent passing gas. Another way is for the patient to insert her finger in the vagina and try to squeeze it using her vaginal muscles. The patient should feel the pressure over her finger and also the sensation in her vagina. Men can be taught in a similar fashion with a finger in the rectum.

Once recognition of the "correct" group of muscles is assured, PFMT sessions can be started. There are many PFMT protocols that are proved to be successful. A number of studies including one by Siu et al.,[9] have demonstrated a considerable success using a program of 30 contractions repeated 3 times daily. During the session, the patient is asked to perform few flicks or 2-to3-second contractions, followed by one sustained (5 second or more) contraction, followed by relaxation of at least 10 seconds. As part of urge control process, and as the patient feels the urge to urinate, the patient is instructed to relax his/her body, start five short PFM contractions, and focus on these muscles. This suppresses the feeling of urgency and the patient has enough time to reach the bathroom while walking in a normal pace. PFMT needs lifelong patient compliance in order to maintain good outcome.

Use of absorbent products (pantiliners, pads, diapers, etc.): This is the first management option for UI in frail, elderly population with other physical and cognitive impairments. It is also a good choice for patients with occasional leakage of small amounts of urine. These products come in variety of sizes and different materials. Some have ingredients that turn to gel when wet, adding more protection. Others have built in deodorants to minimize urine smell. The main purpose is to keep the patient's body dry, avoid urine–skin contact-related complications and makes the urine leakage undetectable by others, and hence minimizes the UI-related emotional and psychological complications.

ROLE OF PHARMACOTHERAPY

Drug Therapy

The major role of drug therapy in UI is in treatment of UUI and MUI. So far, there are no available FDA-approved medications that assure urethral closure and can treat SUI. The most commonly used medications in treatment of UI include the following:

Antimuscarinic Medications

These act by blocking the action of Ach. These medications affect the muscarinic receptors in the bladder as well as other organs resulting in a variety of side effects with constipation and dry mouth being the most common. There are six currently available antimuscarinic medications in the United States. Namely, Oxybutinin, Tolterodine, Trospium, Fesoterodine, Darifenacin, and Solifenacin. They are thought to work through inhibition of bladder sensory innervations as well as detrusor contraction. These medications have proved 70–80% UUI reduction rates. For the best outcome, the use of antimuscarinic medications should be accompanied with behavioral therapy.

There are five different muscarinic receptors (M1-5).[10] M2 and M3 are predominant in the bladder smooth muscle and M3 are considered by Scarpero et al.[11] more important in detrusor contraction; hence, they are thought to be responsible for detrusor overactivity and bladder emptying. M1 receptors are cognition receptors, M2 receptors have a role in heart rate regulation, M3 receptors mediate salivary secretion and bowel movement, M4 receptors are mainly found in the brainstem while their function is unknown, and M5 receptors have a role in accommodation. Antimuscarinics' side effects will be related to their effects on these different receptors. Drugs which can cross the blood brain barrier and affect M1 receptors will induce cognitive impairment, those which block M2 receptors will have a negative impact on the heart rate. Antimuscarinics that block M3 receptors will cause dry mouth and constipation as their main side effects.[12]

Response to antimuscarinic treatment is very subjective. There is no cut-off definition for successful outcome. Success depends mainly on patient perception of symptoms' improvement. Treatment outcome is affected by other confounders that should be considered when counseling patients. These confounders include type of incontinence (UUI vs. MUI), patient lifestyle (amount of fluid the patient drinks every day), associated medical condition (e.g. congestive heart failure), and other medications (e.g. diuretics, bladder irritants, and alpha agonists).

Patient compliance for the medication markedly affects the outcome. Many factors affect patient compliance and should be taken in consideration at time of drug prescription. Factors that affect patient compliance include drug tolerance, cost (along with insurance regulations), mode of delivery, dose frequency, patient age, other comorbidities, severity of symptoms, and treatment outcome. For best results, an open and detailed discussion should be initiated between the physician and the patient before starting treatment. In a survey of 5,392 patients with OAB, 24.5% reported discontinuing 1 antimuscarinic prescription medication or more during the prior 12 months. Survey responses of those who discontinued showed that the most frequently reported reason for discontinued medication was "didn't work as expected."[13] Hence, patients should be counseled that improvement of symptoms is usually perceived 2–3 weeks after initiation of the therapy. Cost and insurance issues should be addressed before drug prescription. Patients other comorbidities should be also considered.

Based on their chemical structure, the antimuscarinics are divided to two major subgroups; tertiary and quaternary amines. All antimuscarinics, except for Trospium are tertiary amines. Tertiary amines are readily absorbable while quaternary amines have lower gastrointestinal absorption and therefore need be taken on an empty stomach. Trospium is the considered the safest in polypharmacy patients because it has the least potential for drug–drug interaction. Trospium and darifenacin have lower tendency for CNS side effects.

β3 agonists (Mirabegron)

Mirabegron is a β3-adrenoceptor agonist which has recently been approved by the FDA for treatment of OAB. The medication acts through a different mechanism of action from that of the antimuscarinic medications. It activates the β3 (the most potent of the β) receptor sin the bladder wall). This results in detrusor muscle relaxation. The medication has also been approved in Japan, Canada and Europe, for the treatment of OAB symptoms. The treatment can be initiated with a starting dose of 25 mg which can be increased to 50 mg daily according to patient response and tolerability.[14]

Estrogen Therapy

This is a well-known treatment strategy for menopause-associated symptoms including hot flashes, vaginal dryness, and night sweats. In menopausal and postmenopausal women, estrogen deficiency has been also proposed as a cause for UTIs, POP, urgency, frequency, and UUI.[15] Estrogen and progesterone receptors are found in vaginal epithelium as well as urethra and bladder trigone.[16] It has been stated by the American College of Obstetricians and Gynecologists that "for genitourinary symptoms associated with menopause, estrogen and progestin have been shown to be beneficial." A recent Cochrane review, however, concluded that treatment with estrogen alone was associated with perceived improvement or cure compared with placebo but that larger trials were needed.

In a recent large, randomized clinical trial by Hendrix et al.[17] estrogen therapy was not found beneficial for treating UI. On the contrary, it was found to precipitate UI in continent women who used estrogen therapy versus placebo. For lower genitourinary only symptoms, local (vaginal) estrogen therapy is preferable. The vaginal estrogen delivery forms available in the United States include estradiol creams (Estrace and Premarin), estradiol vaginal tablets (Vagifem), and estradiol vaginal rings (Estring). The effect is perceived within 4–6 weeks (2–3 weeks for vaginal rings).

Side effects of local estrogen therapy include vaginal discharge, headache, sexual changes, leucorrhea, breast tenderness, vaginal spotting, abdominal pain, nausea, and vomiting. Contraindications for estrogen therapy include hypercoagulable states, history of cardiovascular disease (deep vein thrombosis, strokes, and pulmonary embolism), breast cancer, and/or endometrial cancer. Estrogen should be also used with caution in elderly population because of risk of dementia. Proper instructions should be given to patients regarding risks, benefits, and side effects. Modes of drug delivery (better written) instructions should be also provided.

Other Medical Therapies

Desmopressin Acetate (DDAVP)

These can be used with caution for treatment of nocturia and nocturnal enuresis.[18] Hyponatremia is a major side effect and sodium level should be monitored during therapy.

Tricyclic Antidepressants

These are thought to have anticholinergic and alpha adrenergic properties. Imepramine is usually used for treatment of nocturnal enuresis in both children and adults. However, no studies are available about its use in adults. Furthermore, its use in adults is not FDA approved for treating nocturnal enuresis.

Alpha Agonists

These propose to increase the bladder outlet resistance through activation of the alpha receptors at the urethral smooth muscles and hence improving SUI. The use of these medications is associated with multiple cardiovascular side effects related to their alpha receptor stimulating properties.

Use of Absorbent Products (Pantiliners, Pads, Diapers, etc.)

This is the first management option for UI in frail, elderly population with other physical and cognitive impairments. It is also a good choice for patients with occasional leakage of small amounts of urine. These products come in variety of sizes and different materials. Some have ingredients that turn to gel when wet adding more protection. Others have built in deodorants to minimize urine smell. The main purpose is to keep the patient's body dry, avoid urine-skin contact–related complications and makes the urine leakage undetectable by others and hence minimizes the UI-related emotional and psychological complications.

■ OUTLINE OF SOME PHARMACOTHERAPEUTIC AGENTS[19,20]

Antimuscarinic and Musculotropic Drugs

Propantheline (Pro-Banthine)

Properties: Propantheline is a nonselective (M_1, M_2, and M_3) muscarinic receptor antagonist. It competitively blocks acetylcholine binding to neuroeffector site on detrusor muscle and other muscarinic receptors sites including ganglia.

Indications: Overactive bladder, adult enuresis.

Side effects: Dry mouth, constipation, abdominal discomfort, palpitation, and arrhythmias, CNS stimulation including convulsion, reduced sweating, difficulty micturition and urinary retention, photosensitivity, and allergic reaction.

Contraindication: Glaucoma, urinary retention, bladder outflow obstruction, gastrointestinal atony, and abstruction, ulcerative colitis.

Caution: Cardiac, renal, and hepatic impairment; hyperthyroidism; elderly, reflux esophagitis; pregnancy; breastfeeding.

Interaction: Wide interaction with drugs having parasympathomimetic and antimuscarinic actions. Please determine interaction with any concomitantly administered drug.

Dosage: Propantheline (Pro-Banthine)—15 mg 3 times daily and 30 mg at bed time adjusted according to response to a maximum of 120 mg daily.

Preparation: Oral.

Oxybutinin

Properties: An antimuscarinic drug with high affinity for M_1 and M_3 receptors. It is indicated in patients with urinary frequency, bladder overactivity, bladder instability, nocturnal enuresis, and postoperative bladder spasms.

Side effect: See propantheline.

Contraindications: See propantheline.

Caution: See propantheline.

Dosage: Oxybutinin hydrochloride, oral 2.5 mg 2 to 4 times daily. Elderly 2.5 mg twice daily to a maximum of 5 mg twice daily.

Preparations: Oral—immediate release.

  Oral–modified (extended) release for daily doing, transdermal and intravesical.

Propiverine

Properties: This drug is an antimuscarinic and calcium antagonist. It is indicated in patients with frequency, overactive bladder, neurogenic bladder instability, and postoperative bladder spasms.

Side effects: See propantheline.

Contraindications: Children, also see propantheline.

Caution: See propantheline.

Interaction: See propantheline.

Dosage: Propiverine hydrochloride—15 mg 1–3 times daily

Preparation: Oral

Tolterodine

Properties: Tolterodine is a nonselective antimuscarinic agent. Tolterodine and its metabolites do not cross blood-brain barrier and the drug has low CNS system toxicity. It is indicated in patients with urinary frequency, overactive bladder, and postoperative bladder spasms.

Side effects: See propantheline. Also, fatigue, chest pain, peripheral edema, xerophthalmia, and paresthesia.

Contraindications: See propantheline, children.

Caution: See propantheline

Interaction: See propantheline

Dosage: Oral, 2 mg twice daily may reduce to 1 mg twice daily to minimize side effects.

Preparation: Oral, tolterodine tartrate immediate release.
 – Oral modified (extended)—release for once daily dosing.

Trospium Chloride

Properties: This quaternary amine is a nonselective muscarinic antagonist. It is as effective as oxybutinin with better tolerability. It does not cross blood-brain barrier. Its profile of side effects, contraindications, and interactions are similar to tolterodine.

Dosage: Oral trospium chloride 20 mg twice daily.

Darifenacin

Properties: An antimuscarinic drug with high affinity for M_3 receptors. It is indicated in patients with urinary frequency, bladder overactivity, bladder instability, nocturnal enuresis, and postoperative bladder spasms.

Dosage: Adult over 18 years: 7.5 mg twice daily.

Botulinum A Toxin (Botox)

Properties: Botulinum toxin A blocks acetylecholine release at cholinergic synapses. Inhibition lasts from weeks to 3 to 4 months. The nerves recover only following sprouting. It is indicated in neurogenic detrusor overactivity.

Side effects: Distant muscle jitter, misplaced injection site, muscle paralysis, distant muscles paralysis, injection site burning sensation, allergic reaction, formation of antibodies to Botulinum A toxin, and fever.

Contraindication: Pregnancy, breastfeeding, and disorders of muscle activity

Interaction: Effect enhanced by aminoglycosides and nondepolarizing muscle relaxants.

Dosage: Botulinum A toxin injections, cystoscopic, at 20–30 sites within detrusor but excluding the trigone. Please see manufacturers guide for details.

Desmopressin (DDAVP)

Properties: Desmopressin or 1-deamino-8-D-arginine vasopressin (DDAVP) is an antidiuretic peptide. It acts on V_2 receptors causing water conservation. Desmopressin is indicated for primary nocturnal enuresis in children. This peptide is quickly inactivated by trypsin on oral administration (only 0.15% absorbed).

Side effects: Desmopressin has little V_1-receptor-mediated vascular pressor or gastrointestinal side effects. Its major V_2-receptor-mediated side effect is water intoxication. Other side effects are headache, abdominal pain, nausea, and local effects on nasal passages (edema, rhinorrhea, epistaxis rhinitis, and ulceration) flowing nasal administration.

Contraindications: Renal failure, cardiac insufficiency, and other medical conditions requiring diuresis.

Caution: Excessive fluid intake, elderly, children below 7 years.

Interaction: Diuretic effect potentiated by carbamazepine, chlorpropamide, morphine, NSAIDs, and attenuated by ethanol.

Dosage: Oral: Desmopressin, oral—100–200 µg at bed time starting with lower doses and increasing only if not effective. Withdraw for one week and reassess after 3 months.

Intranasal: Desmopressin, intranasal 10–20 µg at bed time, also withdraw for 1 week and reassess following 3 months of treatment.

REFERENCES

1. Abrams P, Cardozo L, Fall M, et al. The standardisation of terminology of lower urinary tract function: report from the Standardisation Sub-committee of the International Continence Society. Neurourol Urodyn. 2002;21(2):167–78.
2. Garcia JA, Crocker J, Wyman JF, Krissovich M. Breaking the cycle of stigmatization: managing the stigma of incontinence in social interactions. J Wound Ostomy Continence Nurs. 2005;32(1):38–52.
3. Landefeld CS, Bowers BJ, Feld AD, et al. National Institutes of Health state-of-the-science conference statement: prevention of fecal and urinary incontinence in adults. Ann Intern Med. 2008;148(6):449–58.
4. Lifford KL, Curhan GC, Hu FB, Barbieri RL, Grodstein F. Type 2 diabetes mellitus and risk of developing urinary incontinence. J Am Geriatr Soc. 2005;53(11):1851–57.
5. Burgio KL, Goode PS, Urban DA, et al. Preoperative biofeedback assisted behavioral training to decrease post-prostatectomy incontinence: a randomized, controlled trial. J Urol. 2006;175(1):196–201; discussion.
6. Diokno AC, Sampselle CM, Herzog AR, et al. Prevention of urinary incontinence by behavioral modification program: a randomized, controlled trial among older women in the community. J Urol. 2004;171(3):1165–71.

7. Shamliyan TA, Kane RL, Wyman J, Wilt TJ. Systematic review: randomized, controlled trials of nonsurgical treatments for urinary incontinence in women. Ann Intern Med. 2008;148(6):459–73.
8. Leriche B, Conquy S. [Guidelines for rehabilitation management of non-neurological urinary incontinence in women]. Prog Urol. 2010;(Suppl 2):S104-S108.
9. Siu LS, Chang AM, Yip SK. Compliance with a pelvic muscle exercise program as a causal predictor of urinary stress incontinence amongst Chinese women. Neurourol Urodyn. 2003;22(7):659–63.
10. Abrams P, Andersson KE, Buccafusco JJ, et al. Muscarinic receptors: their distribution and function in body systems, and the implications for treating overactive bladder. Br J Pharmacol. 2006;148(5):565–78.
11. Scarpero HM, Dmochowski RR. Muscarinic receptors: what we know. Curr Urol Rep. 2003;4(6):421–8.
12. Wein AJ. Pharmacological agents for the treatment of urinary incontinence due to overactive bladder. Expert Opin Investig Drugs. 2001;10(1):65–83.
13. Schabert VF, Bavendam T, Goldberg EL, Trocio JN, Brubaker L. Challenges for managing overactive bladder and guidance for patient support. Am J Manag Care. 2009;15(4 Suppl):S118-S22.
14. Nitti VW, Khullar V, van Kerrebroeck P, et al. Mirabegron for the treatment of overactive bladder: a prespecified pooled efficacy analysis and pooled safety analysis of three randomized, double-blind, placebo-controlled, phase III studies. Int J Clin Pract. 2013;67(7):619-32.
15. Cardozo L, Lose G, McClish D, Versi E. A systematic review of the effects of estrogens for symptoms suggestive of overactive bladder. Acta Obstet Gynecol Scand. 2004;83(10):892–7.
16. Ballagh SA. Vaginal hormone therapy for urogenital and menopausal symptoms. Semin Reprod Med. 2005;23(2):126–40.
17. Hendrix SL, Cochrane BB, Nygaard IE, et al. Effects of estrogen with and without progestin on urinary incontinence. JAMA. 2005;293(8):935–48.
18. van Kerrebroeck P, Rezapour M, Cortesse A, et al. Desmopressin in the treatment of nocturia: a double-blind, placebo-controlled study. Eur Urol. 2007;52(1):221–9.
19. British National Formulary. BMJ and RPS, London 2008 56:445–8.
20. Griffin ST, Tunner WH. Urinary incontinence. In: Eardley I, Whelan P, Kirby R, Schaeffer A (Eds). Drug treatment in urology. Blackwell, Oxford, UK 2006: 3–20.

CHAPTER 5
Benign Prostatic Hyperplasia

Ismaila A Mungadi, Olayiwola B Shittu, Abdullahi Abdulwahab-Ahmed

■ INTRODUCTION

The frequency of surgery for benign prostatic hyperplasia (BPH) and lower urinary tract symptoms (LUTS) is declining due to increasing success of drug treatment of these conditions. Significant clinical outcome can be obtained with medical treatment without the potential complications of surgery. This has led to a reduction in the number of prostatectomies in different parts of the word.[1,2] The outcome of drug treatment should be compared with standard procedures like transurethral resection. The drugs in current use are aimed at decreasing the dynamic resistance or reducing the prostatic size. In recent times, there is resurgence in the application of various phytotherapeutic agents in the management of patients with LUTS secondary to BPH.

Benign prostatic hyperplasia is a result of prostatic glandular epithelial and fibromuscular hyperplasia. Bladder outlet obstruction secondary to BPH is caused by passive and active urethral resistance. Passive urethral resistance is contributed by hyperplastic stromal elements, epithelial elements, and prostatic capsules. The prostatic smooth muscles controlled by adrenergic nervous system contribute active urethral resistance. Smooth muscles account for about 40% of the area density of hyperplastic prostate.[3] The $α_1$-adrenergic receptors are the most abundant in human prostatic smooth muscles. Antagonist to $α_1$-adrenoceptors can reduce urethral resistance and relieve symptoms of BPH. Although the direct role of androgen in the etiology of BPH is not clear, withdrawal of androgen effect on prostatic cells lead to apoptosis. Testosterone is converted to dihydrotestosterone (DHT) through the action of α-reductase. DHT binds to androgen receptors and the DHT, and receptor complex interact with nuclear DNA leading to transcriptional events and protein synthesis. This process is blocked by 5α-reductase inhibitors. The predominant 5α-reductase enzyme in the prostatic tissue is type 2.

The response of the bladder to BPH and obstruction also contribute to LUTS. These are detrusor instability (which leads to frequency and urgency) and reduced detrusor contractility (which leads to hesitancy, intermittency, and increased residual urine).

Benign Prostatic Hyperplasia

In the elderly, other factors may influence bladder response and contribute to LUTS. These are detrusor aging, primary bladder pathology, neurogenic disease, and polyuria.

The aims of drug treatment are reduction in prostatic size, reduction in dynamic resistance, and improvement in detrusor function. Deterioration of detrusor function is secondary and tends to improve, once the outlet obstruction is relieved. Patients presenting with complicated BPH are not suitable for drug treatment. The efficacy of medical therapy can be assessed using international prostate symptoms score (IPSS)[4] (Table 5.1), and uroflowmetric study.

ALPHA-ADRENERGIC ANTAGONIST

Contraction of the smooth muscles of the prostatic stroma, capsule, and bladder neck is mediated via α_1-adrenergic receptors. Of the three subtypes (α_{1A}, α_{1B}, α_{1D}), α_{1A} is the most predominant in the prostatic smooth muscles. Alpha adrenergic blockade will therefore lead to relaxation of prostatic smooth muscles thus relieving dynamic bladder neck obstruction. Alpha-adrenoceptor blockage may also relieve detrusor over activity by direct effect on the bladder or spinal cord.[5] Alpha-adrenoceptor blockage is more likely to relieve irritative symptoms and has only modest effect on obstructive symptoms. Nonselective α blockers like phenoxybenzamine are effective but have limited application due to their excessive cardiovascular side effects, related to α_2 blockade. Prazosin is a selective α_1 blocker originally used as an antihypertensive. Doxazosin, alfuzosin, silodosin, and terazosin have fewer side effects and allow once daily dosing. Tamsulosin exhibits more specificity against α_{1a} receptor than other α_1 receptor antagonist in current use. These alpha blockers are of proven efficacy in the treatment of BPH and in reducing the risk of urinary retention. The clinical response is rapid. In patients with acute retentions, alpha blockers significantly increase the possibility of spontaneous voiding within 24–48 hours of indwelling catheter removal. They can safely be used in the elderly and can lower blood pressure in patients with coexisting hypertension. Alpha adrenergic blockers do not reduce size of prostate and prevent acute urinary retention.[6]

5-ALPHA REDUCTASE INHIBITORS

Alpha reductase inhibition is the only androgen suppression considered here. Other drugs have not achieved similar level of tolerance and acceptability. Finasteride is a competitive 5-α reductase type 2 inhibitor. It lowers serum and intraprostatic DHT level up to 65–70% and 85–90%, respectively[7] by competing with the enzyme, 5-α reductase, responsible for the conversion of testosterone to the more active DHT. Absence of DHT leads to apoptosis of prostatic cells. Finasteride reduces prostatic size and is indicated in patients with large

Benign Urological Diseases

Table 5.1 International prostate symptom score (IPSS)

Name			Date					
	Not at all	Less than 1 time in 5	Less than half the time	About half the time	More than half the time	Almost always	Your score
Incomplete emptying Over the past month, how often have you had a sensation of not emptying your bladder completely after you finish urinating?	0	1	2	3	4	5	
Frequency Over the past month, how often have you had to urinate again less than two hours after you finished urinating?	0	1	2	3	4	5	
Intermittency Over the past month, how often have you found you stopped and started again several times when you urinated?	0	1	2	3	4	5	
Urgency Over the last month, how difficult have you found it to postpone urination?	0	1	2	3	4	5	
Weak stream Over the past month, how often have you had a weak urinary stream?	0	1	2	3	4	5	
Straining Over the past month, how often have you had to push or strain to begin urination?	0	1	2	3	4	5	

	None	1 time	2 times	3 times	4 times	5 times or more	Your score
Nocturia Over the past month, many times did you most typically get up to urinate from the time you went to bed until the time you got up in the morning?	0	1	2	3	4	5	

Total IPSS score

Quality of life due to urinary symptoms	Delighted	Pleased	Mostly satisfied	Mixed– about equally satisfied and dissatisfied	Mostly dissatisfied	Unhappy	Terrible
If you were to spend the rest of your life with your urinary condition the way it is now, how would you feel about that?	0	1	2	3	4	5	6

Total score: 0-7 Mildly symptomatic; 8-19 moderately symptomatic; 20-35 severely symptomatic.

prostatic gland. It reduces progression of BPH. It produces improvement over a period of several months as against $α_1$-adrenergic blockade. Finasteride is, therefore, only appropriate in patients with large prostate not responding to α-adrenergic antagonist or where α-adrenergic antagonist are contraindicated. Finasteride is effective in reducing gross and recurrent hematuria secondary to BPH and post-prostatectomy. It delays the occurrence of symptoms progression and urinary retention in patients with BPH.

Dutasteride is a 5-α reductase inhibitor that blocks both type 1 and 2 enzymes. Type 1 enzyme is found in the liver and skin. By additional block on type 1 enzyme, dutasteride further reduces serum levels of DHT and is, therefore, more efficacious than finasteride.

■ COMBINATION THERAPY

The combination of an α-adrenergic antagonist and 5-α reductase inhibitor is an attractive therapy. An α-adrenergic antagonist will provide prompt symptomatic relief while the α-reductase inhibitor will alter the disease progression and the natural history of acute retention. Some studies did not confirm direct additive effects but more recent consensus opinion from combination of Avodart (dutesteride) and Tamsulosin study (CombAT) and other randomized case-control studies establish the benefits of combination of 5-α reductase inhibitors and $α_1$ blockers with relief of LUTS from dynamic effect of $α_1$ blockers and long-term effect of 5-α reductase inhibitors on static components leading to overall better outcome on voiding and low incidence of AUR.[8,9] The role of combination therapy is now fully defined in management of BPH. It is better than monotherapy in large gland and in preventing acute urinary retention (AUR). Many urologists now reserve it for initial period of therapy before the full therapeutic effect of 5-α reductase inhibitor is established and in large prostate gland. The cost of such combination must also be taken into consideration.

■ PHYTOTHERAPEUTIC AGENTS

These are agents extracted from the bark, roots, seeds, leaves, flowers, or fruits of plants found in different parts of the world. The extracts are widely available and they are widely used by men. They are known to have significant clinical response in patients with BPH and LUTS. Their mechanism of action is difficult to elucidate and an extract may contain several active components. Extracts are known to have 5-α reductase activity, anti-inflammatory effects, and growth factors modulating activity. Meaningful scientific discussion on these agents is difficult because the extracts are not qualitatively and quantitatively standardized. Some phytotherapeutic agents are, however, listed at the end of this chapter.

OUTLINE OF PHARMACOTHERAPY FOR BPH[10-12]

Alpha 1 Receptor Antagonist

Prazosin

Properties: It is a selective $α_1$ receptor antagonist with similar potencies on $α_{1A}$, $α_{1B}$, and $α_{1D}$ subtypes. It blocks not only $α_1$ receptor in the prostate and bladder neck but arterioles and veins leading to reduced vascular resistance and venous return. Prazosin is well absorbed orally. It is metabolized in the liver and excreted by the kidney. Prazosin has a plasma half-life of 2–3 hours and duration of action of 7 to 10 hours necessitating twice daily dosing.

Side effect: First-dose effect (marked hypotension and syncope 30–90 minutes after initial dose), headache, dizziness, asthenia, depression, dry mouth, nausea, vomiting, constipation, diarrhea, tachycardia, palpitations, and hypersensitivity.

Contraindication: Postural hypotension, micturition syncope.

Caution: Elderly, hepatic impairment, use of antihypertensives.

Interaction: Widely interacts to enhance hypotensive effect of all hypotensive agents including alcohol, angiotensin II antagonist, anesthetic agents, alprostadil, antidepressants, β-blockers, anxiolytic, diuretics, calcium channel blockers, muscle relaxants, and vardenafil.

Dosage: Prazosin (minipress, others) oral start with 0.5 mg twice daily for 3–7 days, adjust according to response to a maximum of 2 mg twice daily. First dose should be taken at bed time and patients must be warned about first-dose effect (see above). Patient should remain lying down until there is no risk of first-dose effect or symptoms abate.

Terazosin

Properties: It is an $α_1$ receptor antagonist. It blocks $α_{1A}$, $α_{1B}$, and $α_{1D}$ subtypes. Terazosin is less potent then prazosin. Terazosin, also, induces apoptosis in prostatic smooth muscle cells, an effect attributable to quinazoline moiety. The half-life is about 12 hours and the duration of action is greater than 18 hours, which permits once daily dose schedule.

Side effects: See prazosin: Also dyspnea, thrombocytopenia, decreased libido, paresthesia.

Contraindication: See prazosin.

Caution: See prazosin.

Interaction: See prazosin.

Dosage: Terazosin (Hytrin, others) initially 1 mg at bedtime, may be doubled at 1 to 2 weeks interval to a maximum of 10 mg daily (usually dose 5–10 mg daily). First dose should be taken at bedtime and patient should be warned about first-dose effect (see above). Patient should remain lying down until there is no risk of first dose effect or symptoms.

Doxazosin

Properties: Highly selective $α_1$ antagonist without distinction between $α_{1A}$, $α_{1B}$, and $α_{1D}$ subtypes. Half-life is about 20 hours and duration may last up to 36 hours. Doxazosin also has apoptosis inducing action on prostatic smooth muscle cells that may be beneficial in the long-term management of BPH. This action is attributable to the quinazoline moiety and is independent of $α_1$ receptor antagonism.

Side effects: See prazosin.

Contraindications: See prazosin.

Caution: See prazosin.

Interaction: See prazosin.

Dosage: Doxazosin (Cardura, others) oral initially 1 mg daily, may be doubled weekly to a maximum of 8 mg daily (usual dose 2–4 mg daily).

First-dose effect: See prazosin.

■ Alfuzosin

Properties: Alfuzosin is an $α_1$ receptor antagonist with no distinction between the $α_{1A}$, $α_{1B}$, and $α_{1D}$ subtypes. It has a half-life of 3 to 5 hours and a slow release preparation is necessary for daily administration.

Side effects: See prazosin. Also chest pain.

Contraindication: See prazosin.

Caution: See prazosin.

Interaction: See prazosin.

Dosage: Alfuzosin (Xatral) intermediate release 2.5–3 mg 3 times daily maximum 10 mg daily.
Alfuzosin (Xatral XL) slow release—10 mg once daily.
First-dose effect: See prazosin.

Silodosin

Properties: Selectively antagonizes $α(1A)$-adrenergic receptors in the prostate and urethra.

Side effects: Abnormal ejaculation, also see prazosin.

Contraindications: See prazosin.

Caution: See prazosin.

Interaction: See prazosin.

Dosage: 4–8 mg daily.

Tamsulosin

Properties: Tamsulosin is an α_1 receptor antagonist with selectivity for α_{1A} and α_{1D} subtypes. This α_{1A} selectivity is responsible for its specificity for prostatic α_1 receptors and minimal effect on blood pressure. Tamsulosin has a half-life of about 5–10 hours.

Side effects: Abnormal ejaculation, also see prazosin.

Contraindications: See prazosin.

Caution: See prazosin.

Interaction: See prazosin.

Dosage: Tamsulosin (Flowmax, others) oral, capsules -0.4 mg daily.

5-Alpha Reductase Inhibitors

Finasteride

Properties: Finasteride is a type 2, 5-α reductase inhibitor. It blocks conversion of testosterone to DHT in the prostate and external genitalia leading to reduced serum and prostatic levels of DHT. Several months may be required before clinical effect manifests. Finasteride reduces prostatic volume and improves urinary flow rate and obstructive symptoms. The drug is also licensed for use in male pattern baldness. It reduces serum levels of prostate specific antigen (PSA) and reference range must be adjusted in patients on finasteride. Finasteride is excreted in significant amount in semen to affect sex partner.

Side effects: Infrequent but include breast tenderness, gynecomastia, decreased libido, impotence, and ejaculatory dysfunction.

Contraindications: Children, adolescents, and women of childbearing age.

Caution: Use condom if partner pregnant or still childbearing, evaluation for prostatic cancer using PSA.

Interaction: No clinically significant interaction reported.

Dosage: Finasteride (Proscar, others) oral—5 mg daily

Dutasteride

Properties: Type I and 2, 5-α reductase antagonist. It leads to rapid lowering of serum DHT and prostate volume shrinkage than achievable with finasteride.

Its clinical efficacy is, however, similar to finasteride and requires several months. Also, excreted in semen to a significant concentrator to affect sex partner.

Side effects: See finasteride.

Contraindications: See finasteride.

Caution: See finasteride.

Interaction: Serum concentration increased by calcium channel blockers such as verapamil.

Dosage: Dutasteride (Avodart) oral, capsule—0.5 mg daily.

Phytotherapeutic Agents

The properties of phytotherapeutic agents is very complex and not fully characterized. The doses are also not standardized. The origin of some extract is listed below. Interested readers are referred to relevant literature for details.

1. Pygeum africanum (African plum)
2. Serenoa repens or Sebal serrulatum (American dwarf palm)
3. Hypoxis rooperi (South African star grass)
4. Cucurbita pepo (Punkin seeds)
5. Pinus (Pine)
6. Picea (Spruce)
7. Urtica dioica (Stinging nettle)

■ REFERENCES

1. Health care financing Administration: BESS Data Washinton DC, 1998.
2. Hotgrewe HL. Current trends in the management of men with lower urinary tract symptoms and benign prostatic hyperplasia. Urology. 1998;51(Suppl A):1–7.
3. Shapiro E, Hatano V, Cepor H. The response of L alpha blockage in benign prostate hyperplasia is related to the percent area density of prostate smooth muscles. Prostate. 1992;21:297–307.
4. Barry MJ, Fowler FJ Jr, O'Leary MP, et al. The American Urological Association Symptom Index for benign prostatic hyperplasia. J Urol. 1992;148:1549–57.
5. Broten T, Scoh A, Siegl PKS, Forray C. Alpha-adrenoceptor blockade inhibits detrusor instability in rats with bladder outlet obstruction. FASEB J. 1998;12:A445.
6. McConnell JD, Roehrborn CG, Bautista O, et al. The Long-term effect of doxazosin, finasteride, and combination therapy on the clinical progression of benign prostatic hyperplasia. N Engl J Med. 2003;349:2387–98.
7. Bartsch G, Rittmaster RS, Klocker H. Dihydrotestosterone and the concept of 5 alpha-reductase inhibition in human benign prostatic hyperplasia. Euro Urol. 2000;37:367–80.

8. Roehrborn CG, Siami P, Barkin J, et al. The effects of combination therapy with dutasteride and tamsulosin on clinical outcomes in men with symptomatic benign prostatic hyperplasia: 4-year results from the CombAT study. Eur Urol. 2010;57: 123–31.
9. Barkin J, Roehrborn CG, Siami P, et al. Effect of dutasteride, tamsulosin and the combination on patient-reported quality of life and treatment satisfaction in men with moderate-to-severe benign prostatic hyperplasia: 2-year data from the CombAT trial. BJU Int. 2009;103:919–26.
10. British National Formulary. BMJ and RPS, London 2008,56:443–44.
11. Westfall TC, Westfall DP. Adrenergic agonist and antagonist. In: Brunton LL, Lazo JS, Parker KL (Eds). Goodman and Gilman's The pharmacological basis of therapeutics, 11th edn., McGraw-Hill, New-York, NY, 2006:237–95.
12. Schilit S, Benzeroual KE. Silodosin: a selective alpha1A-adrenergic receptor antagonist for the treatment of benign prostatic hyperplasia. Clin Ther. 2009;31: 2489–502.

CHAPTER 6

Medical Treatment of Urolithiasis

Ehab Eltahawy, Ismaila A Mungadi

■ INTRODUCTION

Urolithiasis is a widespread and multifactorial disease of mankind. It has changed in epidemiology over the last century due to changes in socioeconomic profile of various populations.[1] The lifetime risk is about 10–15% in the developed world, but can be as high as 20–25% in the Middle East. Furthermore, the risk of recurrence is 14% at 1 year, 35% at 2 years, and 52% at 10 years after a single episode of a calcium-containing kidney stone.[2]

There is strong evidence that stone formation is linked to metabolic disorders; thus, urologists should realize their role to treat as well as prevent further episodes of stone formation. Grampsas et al.[3] showed that almost all patients, first time and recurrent stone formers, were very interested in finding out why they form kidney stones and were eager to follow a fluid, dietary, and/or drug therapy program to prevent stones in the future. A good working knowledge of the principles of evaluation of kidney stones will help the urologist to be able to formulate a strategy plan for their prevention. Much of the advancement in treatment that led to a decline in morbidity and mortality from stone disease was in the areas of endoscopic and shock wave therapy. Medical therapy to expel stones and to prevent them is evolving.

■ RISK STRATIFICATION

Low-risk population as a first-time stone former may be subjected to a simplified evaluation while individuals who have recurrent stones, or would develop complications from a recurrent episode, should certainly get a more comprehensive workup. These include patients with solitary kidneys, chronic kidney disease, or medical comorbidities. Patients should be considered for testing when they are suspected to have metabolic derangements as morbidly obese, gout, bowel disease, bone disease, renal tubular acidosis (RTA), hyperparathyroidism, or those on calcium supplementation.

Patients with particular surgical difficulty to access their stones may also require metabolic studies as after urinary diversion, or with spine deformities. Other subgroups include children, sensitive jobs as pilots may benefit from this approach.

■ EVALUATION OF NEPHROLITHIASIS

Evaluation starts with history and physical examination. Information is valuable on the patients' dietary habits particularly high salt food, oxalate rich and animal protein, and amount and type of fluid intake, as citrus fluids (tend to prevent stones). Extensive social history on outdoor jobs or in hot environments. Medical history of sarcoidosis, and metabolic syndrome and diabetes have been linked to increased risk of stone formation. Past surgical history of bowel resection predisposes to oxalate stones. Review of prior medications especially those that are linked to increased stone formation, for example, chemotherapy, antiretroviral therapy, carbonic anhydrase inhibitors such as acetazolamide (can induce RTA), furosemide (which can induce hypercalciuria), calcium and vitamin D supplements. It is important to ask about family history of stone disease. There are a number of hereditary diseases associated with stone formation, for example, cysteinuria and primary hyperoxaluria.[4]

Noncontrast helical CT scan provides the best imaging tool for diagnosis, localization, and characterization of urinary stones. Its use is limited by its availability, affordability, and the radiation exposure. It accurately shows the stone volume and orientation in relation to the anatomy of the kidney, which is important for surgical management (percutaneous stone removal). It is useful in identification of uric acid stones. It does not predict kidney function, however, and is less accurate in planning shock wave lithotripsy (SWL). Plain radiographs may be useful in this respect, as they show the density of the stone. Intravenous urography may be useful in planning in some types of urinary calculi. Its use is, however, becoming limited by the need to inject contrast with its inherent risks, and being not suitable for patients with renal impairment. Ultrasound may be useful in particular situations as in pregnant patients. It has low sensitivity in detecting ureteral calculi, Doppler ultrasound with resistive index, and plain X-ray combined with ultrasound may improve its use.

Metabolic workup should be initiated preferably 3–4 weeks after an endoscopic intervention or SWL when all the stones are cleared. Table 6.1 shows the prevalence of metabolic abnormalities on metabolic workup.

Stone analysis is an important part of the evaluation of first-time and recurrent stone formers. Stone composition may direct further evaluation, as it has some predictive value in diagnosing conditions associated with calcium stone formation. Calcium apatite stones and mixed calcium oxalate/calcium apatite stones form in patients with type 1 RTA and hyperparathyroidism.[5]

Medical Treatment of Urolithiasis

Table 6.1: Prevalence of metabolic abnormalities[8]

Metabolic Defect	Prevalence (%)
Hypercalciuria	28–53
Hypocitraturia	10–50
Hyperoxaluria	2–30
Hyperuricosuria	10–40
Gouty diatheses	15–30
Low volume	10–50
Hypomagnesuria	5–10
Cystinuria	< 1

Source: Levy FL, Adams-Huet B, Pak CY. Ambulatory evaluation of nephrolithiasis: an update of a 1980 protocol. Am J Med. 1995;98:50.

All stone formers should get an initial blood test, a urine analysis with culture if infected, as well as stone analysis. Blood testing include kidney function test, electrolytes: sodium, potassium, chloride, serum calcium, and uric acid. Patients with hypercalcemia or high normal serum calcium levels (especially those who form calcium phosphate stones) are subjected to other blood tests, including serum intact parathyroid hormone and phosphate levels.

The simplified approach of history, stone analysis, and serum chemistry studies is recommended for low-risk patients, and 24-hour urine testing is added for the evaluation of high-risk patients. Urine is collected while the patient is consuming a self-selected diet.

Our strategy is to initially have the patient collect a single 24-hour specimen and only proceed with obtaining another if no abnormalities are identified.

Urine volume and pH are determined, and creatinine, calcium, oxalate, citrate, uric acid, sodium, potassium, magnesium, phosphate, and urea nitrogen are measured. Creatinine is measured to assess the accuracy of the collection. Urine volume is an index of hydration. Calcium, oxalate, citrate, uric acid, and pH are measured to detect hypercalciuria, hyperoxaluria, hypocitraturia, hyperuricosuria, gouty diathesis, and the propensity to form calcium phosphate stones. Excretion of sodium and magnesium excretion correlates with their ingestion. Urea nitrogen is a surrogate for total protein consumption. A high proportion of patients with calcium stones have increased calcium excretion. Some groups have advocated supplemental testing to define the cause of hypercalciuria such as determining the response to calcium restriction, fasting, and calcium loading. However, such testing is rarely necessary from a practical standpoint as the initial management would be implementation of dietary modifications and, if this is not successful, administration of a thiazide diuretic or indapamide.

MEDICAL THERAPY

Initial medical management of stones during the episode include controlling pain, infection, chemodissolution, and helping with expulsion of small stones from the ureter. After the acute stone episode, prevention include dietary modifications and pharmacotherapy.

During a Stone Episode

Narcotics such as pethidine give adequate relief from pain but nonsteroidal anti-inflammatory drugs (e.g., Diclofenac sodium, Ibuprofen) are as effective with fewer side effects. A stone less than 0.5 cm in diameter causing partial obstruction is expected to be passed out in 48 hours in 40–50% of cases. A distal and single ureteric stone at the time of diagnosis is more likely to pass spontaneously than a proximal or multiple stones. Stone passage rate can be augmented with medical expulsion therapy[6] using alpha blockers (e.g., tamsulosin, terazosin, or doxazosin) or calcium channel blockers (e.g. nifedipine). The ureterovesical junction is the most common site for stone impaction, however other sites include the ureteropelvic junction and the iliac vessel crossing.

Chemodissolution of Stones

Oral alkalinization therapy to render urine pH to between 6.5 and 7 is successful in dissolving pure uric acid stones. This can be achieved using potassium citrate (60 mEq in three divided doses per day), sodium bicarbonate (3 g every 2 hours until urinary pH is above 7 then 5–10 g daily to maintain alkaline urine), or potassium bicarbonate. Acetazolamide, in a dose of 250 mg 3 times a day, may be used to augment the urinary alkalinizing action of citrate or bicarbonate. It inhibits carbonic anhydrase thereby increasing urinary bicarbonate excretion. This is indicated in kidney lithiasis when the stones are not associated with obstruction, or infection.

After the Stone Episode

Hydration and Diet

Urinary volume is the most important factor in predicting stone recurrence rate.[7]

Reduced dietary calcium consumption, and increased oxalate have been identified as risk factors for developing a kidney stone.[9] The risk associated with reduced calcium consumption has been attributed to increased oxalate absorption and renal excretion. Increased oxalate consumption increases its urinary excretion, and hence forming stones. Metabolic studies have shown that increased sodium consumption augments calcium excretion and reduces citrate excretion.[10] In addition, increased animal protein consumption has been reported to amplify calcium and uric acid excretion, and reduce that of citrate in similar studies.[11]

All calcium stone formers should increase fluid intake to maintain adequate urine volume (>2 l a day for adults) and consume well-balanced meals. Those with hypercalciuria should limit animal protein (<50 g a day) and sodium intake (<100 mEq or 2.3 g a day) while maintaining adequate dietary calcium intake (1 to 1.2 g a day for adults). Individuals with hypocitraturia should limit sodium and animal protein intake, and consume more fruits (especially citrus) and vegetables. The majority of individuals with hyperoxaluria should reduce oxalate consumption: wheat bran, spinach, cocoa, tea, nuts, and vitamin C (<100 mg daily for adults). Consultation with a dietician may also facilitate compliance.

Pharmacotherapy

Patients who do not respond to dietary therapy or in whom a more aggressive approach is needed initially are candidates for pharmacologic therapy. Dietary modifications should be continued as they may improve response to pharmacologic intervention.

Hypercalciuria

Calcium stones formers whose urinary calcium excretion is below the threshold of hypercalciuria may benefit from an approach to reduce calcium excretion. Randomized, controlled prospective trials assessing the efficacy of thiazide therapy showed reduced stone activity in those patients who did not have hypercalciuria.[12]

Level 1 evidence exists demonstrating that thiazide therapy reduces the incidence of recurrent stone events. In a Cochrane meta-analysis of four randomized prospective trials, thiazide therapy with some form of dietary modification was compared solely to dietary modification.[13] Thiazide therapy resulted in a 61% reduction in stone recurrence and an 18% decrease in stone formation rate (stones per patient per year).

The current proposed mechanism for the hypocalciuric action of thiazide diuretics is that they inhibit sodium reabsorption in the distal convoluted tubule, promoting sodium and water loss, and resulting in volume contraction that promotes passive reabsorption of calcium in the proximal tubule leading to its diminished urinary excretion.[14] This action is attenuated by the ingestion of sodium that underscores the importance of limiting its intake. Indapamide, an antihypertensive similar to thiazide, at low dose of 1.5 mg daily was found to reduce hypercalciuria in stone patients by 20–50% with few side effects.[15]

Various doses for adults can be used, and it is best to start at a low dose that can be increased if necessary. Starting doses are 1.25 to 2.5 mg 1 time a day indapamide, 12.5 mg 1 time to 50 mg twice daily hydrochlorothiazide and

25 to 50 mg 1 time a day chlorthalidone. Thiazides can induce hypokalemia and hypocitraturia, and so it may be necessary to prescribe potassium citrate or potassium chloride adjunctively to prevent hypokalemia, intracellular acidosis, and resultant hypocitraturia, considered in patients who do not respond to dietary modifications or are intolerant of thiazide therapy.

Augmenting Citrate Excretion

Hypocitraturia has several etiologies including distal RTA, bowel disturbances, and use of thiazide diuretics, and it may be idiopathic. The therapy of choice for most hypocitraturic calcium oxalate stone formers is potassium citrate, as it increases urine pH and urinary citrate excretion, corrects or improves metabolic acidosis, and inhibits precipitation of calcium oxalate crystals. In addition, potassium citrate reduces the risk of uric acid crystal precipitation, thus attenuating heterogeneous nucleation with calcium oxalate. An added benefit of potassium citrate therapy in individuals with distal RTA is correction of hypokalemia.

The preferred agent for treating hypocitraturia is potassium citrate. The dose for adults is based on the degree of hypocitraturia and associated acidosis. Adults are generally prescribed 20 to 30 mEq twice a day orally but this may need to be adjusted based on urinary citrate response, degree of amelioration of systemic acidosis and urine pH. An increase in pH could theoretically increase the risk of calcium phosphate kidney stone formation. Patients with type 1 RTA may require large doses of potassium citrate to induce a therapeutic response. In such cases a reduction or correction of acidosis, lowering of calcium excretion, and an increase in citrate excretion result but urine pH is typically not altered. Liquid and pill forms of potassium citrate are available. The former is preferred in patients with small bowel issues as gastrointestinal transport time may be accelerated.

Sodium citrate or sodium bicarbonate is used in patients who do not tolerate the potassium preparation, have impaired kidney function to an extent that hyperkalemia is present or may readily ensue, or have high normal to elevated serum potassium levels.

Hyperuricosuric calcium nephrolithiasis may benefit from allopurinol therapy. Allopurinol is a xanthine oxidase inhibitor that blocks conversion of hypoxanthine to xanthine, a uric acid precursor. In a randomized controlled trial 100 mg allopurinol therapy 3 times daily was compared to placebo in hyperuricosuric, normocalciuric calcium oxalate stone formers.[16] Allopurinol significantly decreased the rate of stone recurrence as well as significantly prolonged the interval to stone recurrence. Adult doses range from 100 to 300 mg daily.

Magnesium increases the solubility of calcium, oxalate and phosphate in the urine, and theoretically increases citrate excretion. Hypomagnesuria has been described as a risk factor for stone formation, although this has not been definitively proven. It occurs in only a small percentage of patients, some of whom have coexistent hypocitraturia. Magnesium supplements have been recommended for these patients and include 500 mg twice a day magnesium oxide or magnesium gluconate orally with meals for adults. A common side effect of magnesium supplementation is diarrhea, and so the dose may need to be adjusted based on individual tolerance.

Controlling Oxalate Excretion

In patients who have idiopathic hyperoxaluria, and in those who do not respond to the aforementioned dietary modifications, pyridoxine therapy may be considered. The typical adult dose is 50 to 100 mg daily, and neurotoxicity is a potential side effect. Calcium supplements, preferably calcium citrate, can be administered to those with low normal calcium excretion and has been reported to be an effective method of treating idiopathic hyperoxaluria. Fish oil has been shown to reduce oxalate excretion.[17] Lactic acid bacterial species are known to degrade oxalate, and probiotic formulations have been administered to stone formers with mixed results.[18]

Enteric hyperoxaluria should be suspected in any patient who has an anatomic or functional small bowel problem, or has been subjected to gastric bypass, jejunoileal bypass, biliopancreatic diversion, or other procedures that result in malabsorption. These patients may also have reduced calcium and citrate excretion. They should be placed on a low oxalate, low fat, and normal to increased calcium diet.[19] Calcium supplements, preferably calcium citrate, are administered at the typical initial adult dose of 1 to 2 g 3 times a day orally with meals. The dose is increased if the response is not adequate. Probiotic therapy has been shown to be effective in this patient cohort, with a 19–24% reduction in oxalate excretion.[20] Cholestyramine, an agent that binds bile acids and salts, has been shown to reduce oxalate excretion in these patients. Natural bile acid replacement therapy also decreases urinary oxalate and fecal fat excretion.

Primary hyperoxaluria (PH) should be suspected in any adult with a daily oxalate excretion > 75 mg without evidence of bowel disease or dietary indiscretions, or in children with an oxalate excretion > 1 to 2 mmol per 1.73 m^2. This disease usually manifests during childhood. All patients, regardless of disease type, are treated with pyridoxine. The typical starting dose in children is 5 mg per kg daily, which may be increased to 10 mg per kg daily. Other agents that have been used in these patients are orthophosphates and sodium or potassium citrate. Patients with type 1 PH are at high risk for end-stage renal disease. Those who are not pyridoxine sensitive are candidates for combined hepatic and renal transplant, while patients who are sensitive may be treated effectively with renal transplantation alone.[21]

Gouty Diathesis

The main driver in gouty diathesis is low urine pH. Thus, the goal is to increase urine pH to 6.0 to 6.5. Potassium citrate is the preferred therapy but sodium bicarbonate and sodium citrate are alternatives. The former is favored as the latter two may increase calcium excretion due to the concomitant sodium load.

Struvite Stones

A higher emphasis is placed on the need for intervention and a stone-free result due to the risk of renal failure and death.

Of patients with end-stage renal disease secondary to nephrolithiasis 42% had infection-related struvite stones.[22] The prevalence of struvite stones is higher in patients with neurogenic bladder, including those with spinal cord injuries.[23]

In an 8-year follow-up study of patients who underwent percutaneous nephrolithotomy (PCNL) for staghorn calculi 28% had renal deterioration and the main risk factor was recurrent stones or residual fragments.[24] Furthermore, the risk of death after PCNL for staghorn struvite calculi in 8 years was 0% if the patient was stone-free and 3% if there were residual fragments. Because of these findings, it is recommended that residual fragments should not be left in patients with struvite stones, even if asymptomatic, because of the risks of growth of these stones, renal deterioration, and mortality.

Although antibiotic prophylaxis is commonly prescribed following PCNL for struvite stones, there is no clinical evidence to support this practice. In contrast, studies on acetohydroxamic acid have demonstrated a significant decrease in the risk of residual stone fragments increasing in size. The mechanism of action is by inhibiting bacterial urea hydrolysis and ammonia production. Dose is 250 mg orally 3–4 times daily.

Cystine Stones

Before analysis of calculus composition, the presence of stone disease is often first identified through routine imaging. On plain X-rays cystine stones appear less radiopaque than calcium-containing stones and can sometimes be difficult to identify. The first test performed is often urine microscopy, which can identify the pathognomonic hexagonal crystals, particularly in a first morning void urine sample due to its high concentration and relatively low pH. Crystals are only seen in approximately 25–39% of patients with cystinuria and are never found in normal subjects. Not surprisingly, there are some data that the presence of urinary cystine crystals may correlate with active cystine stone formation, and thus may be a useful tool for monitoring medical management.[25] Cystine supersaturation in urine is volume and pH dependent, with solubility increasing from approximately 250 mg per liter at a pH of 7.0 to 500 mg per liter or more at a pH of 7.5 or greater.[26] As such, a urine cysteine concentration below 250 mg per liter will usually prevent cysteine crystallization and lead to dissolution of existing crystals.

Treatment of patients with cystinuria and cystine stones relies on decreasing cystine urinary supersaturation. Dietary measures, including increasing fluid intake, and restricting sodium and protein consumption, should initially be taken in all affected patients and can be used solely, or more commonly, in combination with medical therapy. The main tenets of medical therapy are to increase cystine solubility by urinary alkalization and with thiol-containing drugs. Patients should be counseled on the need to produce at least 3 l of urine output daily, which may require fluid intake of up to 4 to 5 l a day. Furthermore, it is important that patients drink not only throughout the day, but also at night to ensure sufficient overnight diuresis and to decrease nocturnal aggregation of crystals. Potas per kg daily in 3 to 4 divided doses to achieve adequate urinary alkalization. Medical management with thiol-containing agents may be added to the treatment regimen in those patients who continue to have refractory disease. The two most commonly used thiol-containing drugs are D-penicillamine and mercaptopropionylglycine, also known as tiopronin. In one study, discontinuation of therapy secondary to adverse reactions was as high as 69% in the D-penicillamine group versus 30% in the tiopronin group.[27] Adverse effects include rashes, nausea, vomiting, fever, diarrhea, arthralgias, leukopenia, thrombocytopenia, proteinuria secondary to membranous glomerulonephritis, hepatotoxicity, and vitamin B6 deficiency. Tiopronin can be used as a long-term preventive therapy if well tolerated. Regardless of the thiol-containing drug that is chosen, patients should be periodically monitored with liver enzyme and hematologic studies. Unfortunately, complying with medical management recommendations can be difficult for patients. In one series only 15% of medically treated patients were able to maintain therapeutic success as defined by urine cystine concentrations less than 300 mg per liter.[28]

■ FOLLOW-UP STUDIES

Follow-up studies are recommended to assess response to the prescribed interventions, assess compliance, and monitor for untoward effects. Patients who have solely been prescribed dietary modifications should be evaluated with a 24-hour urine study at 3 to 6 months. If the results are not encouraging, an alternative strategy should be considered such as implementation of medical therapy. If results are satisfactory and stone activity is quiescent, these studies do not need to be repeated unless recurrences develop. Serum electrolytes, calcium, glucose, blood urea nitrogen, and creatinine should be checked 2 to 3 weeks after thiazide diuretics or indapamide is prescribed. If these results are normal, the interval for such testing can be extended to 6 to 12 months. Liver enzymes should be monitored in those who are taking allopurinol before administration, again in 3 to 6 months and yearly thereafter. The 24-hour urine studies in those prescribed medical therapy are repeated at 3 months and, if response is satisfactory, urinalysis is performed yearly thereafter.

■ REFERENCES

1. Blacklock NJ. The epidemiology of renal lithiasis. In urinary calculus disease. Wickham JEA (Ed.), Churchill Livingstone, London, UK, 1979;21–39.
2. Uribarri J, Oh MS, Carroll HJ. The first kidney stone. Ann Intern Med. 1989;111:1006.
3. Grampsas SA, Moore M, Chandhoke PS. 10-year experience with extracorporeal shockwave lithotripsy in the state of Colorado. J Endourol. 2000;14:711–4.
4. Chandhoke PS. Evaluation of the recurrent stone former. Urol Clin N Am. 2007;34:315–22.
5. Kourambas J, Aslan P, Teh CL, et al. Role of stone analysis in metabolic evaluation and medical treatment of nephrolithiasis. J Endourol. 2001;15:181.
6. Sign A, Alter HJ, Littlepage A. A systematic review of medical therapy to facilitate passage of ureteric calculi. Ann Emerg Med. 2007;50:552–63.
7. Pak CY, Sakhaee K, Crowther C, Brinkley L. Evidence justifying a high fluid intake in treatment of nephrolithiasis. Ann Intern Med. 1980;93:36–9.
8. Levy FL, Adams-Huet B, Pak CY. Ambulatory evaluation of nephrolithiasis: an update of a 1980 protocol. Am J Med. 1995;98:50.
9. Curhan GC, Willett WC, Rimm EB, et al. A prospective study of dietary calcium and other nutrients and the risk of symptomatic kidney stones. N Engl J Med. 1993;328:833.
10. Sakhaee K, Harvey JA, Padalino PK, et al. The potential role of salt abuse on the risk for kidney stone formation. J Urol. 1993;150:310.
11. Kok DJ, Iestra JA, Doorenbos CJ, et al. The effects of dietary excesses in animal protein and in sodium on the composition and the crystallization kinetics of calcium oxalate monohydrate in urines of healthy men. J Clin Endocrinol Metab. 1990;71:861.
12. Ettinger B, Citron JT, Livermore B, et al. Chlorthalidone reduces calcium oxalate calculous recurrence but magnesium hydroxide does not. J Urol. 1988;139:679.
13. Escribano J, Balaguer A, Pagone F, et al. Pharmacological interventions for preventing complications in idiopathic hypercalciuria. Cochrane Database Syst Rev. 2009;CD004754.
14. Mensenkamp AR, Hoenderop JG, Bindels RJ. Recent advances in renal tubular calcium reabsorption. Curr Opin Nephrol Hypertens. 2006;15:524.
15. Ceylan K, Topal C, Erkoc R, et al. Effect of indapamide on urinary calcium excretion in patients with and without urinary stone disease. Ann Pharmacother. 2005;39:1034.
16. Ettinger B, Tang A, Citron JT, et al. Randomized trial of allopurinol in the prevention of calcium oxalate calculi. N Engl J Med. 1986;315:1386.
17. Ortiz-Alvarado O, Miyaoka R, Kriedberg C, et al. Omega-3 fatty acids eicosapentaenoic acid and docosahexaenoic acid in the management of hypercalciuric stone formers. Urology. 2012;79:282.

18. Campieri C, Campieri M, Bertuzzi V, et al. Reduction of oxaluria after an oral course of lactic acid bacteria at high concentration. Kidney Int. 2001;60:1097.
19. Nordenvall B, Backman L, Burman P, et al. Low-oxalate, low-fat dietary regimen in hyperoxaluria following jeju- noileal bypass. Acta Chir Scand. 1983;149:89.
20. Lieske JC, Goldfarb DS, De Simone C, et al. Use of a probiotic to decrease enteric hyperoxaluria. Kidney Int. 2005;68:1244.
21. Monico CG, Milliner DS. Combined liver-kidney and kidney-alone transplantation in primary hyperoxaluria. Liver Transpl. 2001;7:954.
22. Jungers P, Joly D, Barbey F, et al. ESRD caused by nephrolithiasis: prevalence, mechanisms, and prevention. Am J Kidney Dis. 2004;44:799.
23. Donnellan SM, Bolton DM. The impact of contemporary bladder management techniques on struvite calculi associated with spinal cord injury. BJU Int. 1999;84:280.
24. Teichman JM, Long RD, Hulbert JC. Long-term renal fate and prognosis after staghorn calculus management. J Urol. 1995;153:1403.
25. Daudon M, Cohen-Solal F, Barbey F, et al. Cystine crystal volume determination: a useful tool in the management of cystinuric patients. Urol Res. 2003;31:207.
26. Goldfarb D, Coe F, Asplin J. Urinary cystine excretion and capacity in patients with cystinuria. Kidney Int. 2006;69:1041.
27. Pak C, Fuller C, Sakhaee K, et al. Management of cysteine nephrolithiasis with mercaptopropionylglycin. J Urol. 1986;136:1003.
28. Pietrow P, Auge B, Weitzer A, et al. Durability of medical management of cystinuria. J Urol. 2003;169:68.

BIBLIOGRAPHY

1. Kidney stones: pathophysiology and medical management: Moe OW, Lancet. 367(2006):333–44.
2. Metabolic evaluation and medical management of the calcium stone former: Lange JN, Mufarrji PW, Wood KD, Assimos DG, AUA Update series. 22;31(2012):222–31.
3. Reconsideration of the 1988 NIH consensus statement on prevention and treatment of kidney stones: are the recommendations out of date? Goldfarb DS, Reviews in Urology. 4;2(2002):53–60.

CHAPTER 7

Miscellaneous Use of Drugs

(Late) Hyacinth N Mbibu, Ismaila A Mungadi

■ PREMATURE EJACULATION

Ejaculation normally occurs during orgasm. It is the consequence of cerebral integration at sexual stimuli resulting in a coordinated response. During orgasm, internal urethral sphincter at the bladder neck closes, external sphincter relaxes, and emission of semen into the bulbous urethra occurs. This is followed by rhythmic contractions of bulbocavernus muscles that force the semen through the urethra (ejaculation).

Premature ejaculation (PE) is the occurrence of ejaculations with minimal sexual stimulation. It is a very subjective symptom but should be considered a problem when orgasm and ejaculations occur in less than a minute of initiation of intercourse and before the man wishes it. The female partner may also be bothered by PEs. PE is mostly psychogenic; therefore, psychotherapy and behavioral therapy should be considered first. Other methods of delaying ejaculations are the use of condom and local anesthetics such as Lidocaine crème at the expense of full sexual pleasure.

Selective serotonin reuptake inhibitors (SSRI) have been proven to be of value in delaying ejaculations in men with PE,[1,2] although not approved in many countries. Drugs such as paroxetine, sertraline, or fluoxetine may be used.

These drugs block neuronal reupstate of serotonin thereby prolonging their synaptic effect. Increased synaptic availability of serotonin stimulates post synaptic 5-HT receptors. Stimulation of 5-HT_3 is suspected to contribute to common side effects including delayed or impaired orgasm.[3] Paroxetine may be used in a dose of 10–20 mg daily or 20 mg 3-4 hours before intercourse.[4] These drugs have a wide range of interactions and side effects, including withdrawal symptoms on prolonged use. Please consult standard pharmacotherapy literature and manufacturers guide before use.

■ PRIAPISM

This is a condition of prolonged painful erection without sexual excitement that may be caused by the following:

Miscellaneous Use of Drugs

- Sickle cell disease
- Leukemia
- Intracavernosal injection of papaverine and other vasoactive medications
- Pelvic tumor
- Spinal cord injury
- Perineal trauma with cavernous artery injury
- Priapism is idiopathic in 40% of cases.

Hemodynamic Classification

Low Flow Priapism (Ischemic or Veno-occlusive)

This is a physiologic obstruction to venous outflow leading to corpora cavernosal congestion with highly viscous, poorly oxygenated and acidotic blood. If not relieved in 4 hours it progresses like a compartment syndrome with ischemia, followed by corpora cavernosal fibrosis and erectile failure. Low flow priapism presents with painful sustained rigid penile erection.

High-Flow Priapism

In high flow the arterial flow continues with oxygenated blood but the venous outflow is normal. High-flow priapism presents with, unprovoked, painless, rigid to partial erection and a history of perineal trauma. Ischemia does not occur and cavernous blood flow continues with high O_2 content and normal CO_2. Patients regain erection following arteriography and appropriate surgical ligation or embolization of ruptured cavernosal artery.

Medical Treatment

There is no medical treatment for high-flow priapism.

The aim of treatment in low-flow priapism is to abort erection as soon as possible and in less than 24 hours to prevent corporal fibrosis and erectile failure.

Corporal aspiration, irrigation, and injection with an adrenergic agonist (e.g. Adrenaline 1:100,000 or phenylephrine 0.25–0.5 mg every 5 minutes) repeated until detumescence occurs.[5] This is effective if started early.

Hydration and oxygenation should be instituted in patient with sickle cell followed by cavernosal aspiration and irrigation. High-flow priapism is a severe urologic emergency; cases not responding to intracavernosal injection should be considered for surgical treatment.

Recurrent priapism in patients with sickle-cell disease may be ameliorated with long-term low-dose sildenafil acting to stabilize corporal smooth muscles and regularize erection.[6,7] Priapism from hematological malignancy is treated by initial general resuscitation and cytotoxic drugs.

INFERTILITY

The World Health Organization defines infertility as the inability of sexually active noncontracepting couple to achieve pregnancy in 1 year.[8] In about 40% of cases the male factor is to blame; in another 40% of cases the female factor and in the remaining cases it is a combination of male and female factors.

Infertility can result from a variety of congenital and acquired urogenital abnormalities, infective causes, endocrine anomalies, genetic abnormalities, and immunological problems. Infertility may be idiopathic in up to 75% cases.

Management of infertility requires proper evaluation of the patient including his female partner. In addition to detailed history and examination several basic laboratory tests, radiologic assessment, and testicular biopsy may be required to determine the cause. Standard semen analysis (Table 7.1) usually forms the basis for important decisions and the need for further andrological testing.[9] If initial evaluation fails to reveal the cause of infertility, specialized testing such as immunologic and genetic analysis may be resorted to.

If a cause for the infertility is evident, it may be found to be pre-testicular, testicular, or post-testicular. Pre-testicular causes are related to hypothalamic and pituitary diseases and may be amenable to drug manipulation. Most testicular and post-testicular diseases are not amenable to drug therapy. Drug therapy for idiopathic infertility is largely empirical with no scientifically proven efficacy.

Table 7.1: Standard value for semen analysis according to the 1999 WHO criteria

Volume	≥ 2.0 ml
pH	7.0–8.0
Sperm concentration	≥ 20 million/ml
Total no. of spermatozoa	≥ 40 million/ejaculate
Motility	≥ 50% with progressive motility
	25% with rapid motility within 60 min after ejaculation
Morphology	≥ 14% of normal shape and form
Viability	> 50% of spermatozoa
Leukocytes	< 1 million/ml
Immunobead test (IBT)	< 50% spermatozoa with adherent particles
MAR (Mixed antiglobia reaction) test	< 50% spermatozoa with adherent particles

Source: World Health Organization. WHO laboratory manual for the examination of human semen and spermcervical mucus interaction, 4th edn. Cambridge University Press, Cambridge, UK, 1999.

Role of Medical Therapy in Infertility

Pyospermia

The source of elevated leukocytes in semen should be investigated in patients with pyospermia. The anatomic site of infection (urethra prostate, and seminal vesicles, epididymics) and possible infecting agent including chlamydia and mycoplasma should be investigated and treated with antibiotics (see Chapter 2). The use of antibiotics is associated with improved sperm function and increased conception rate in patients with pyospermia.[10]

Retrograde Ejaculation

Neurogenic causes, anatomic abnormalities of the urethra, and bladder neck and pharmacological therapy should be ruled out as causes of retrograde ejaculation before medical treatment is considered.

The following drugs could be used to increase resistance at bladder neck and encourage antegrade ejaculation.
- Ephedrine sulfate at a dose of 10–15 mg 4 times daily.
- Imipramine, at 25–50 mg twice daily
- Bromopheniramine maleate 8 mg twice daily.

Hyperprolactinemia

Hyperprolactinemia interferes with gonadotropine-releasing hormone (GnRH) release. Evident prolactin secreting lesions are treated surgically. Nonobvious lesions can be treated with bromocriptine, 5–10 mg daily. This may help to restore pituitary balance.

Hypogonadotrophic Hypogonadism

Patients with Kallmann syndrome do not secrete GnRH that stimulate production of pituitary luteinizing hormone (LH) and follicle-stimulating hormone (FSH). This may be treated with human chorionic gonadotropin (hCG), 1,000–2,000 IU 3 times weekly and FSH (recombinant) 75 1U twice weekly.

In patients with low sperm count and in the setting low-normal LH, FSH, and testosterone; clomiphene therapy may be beneficial.[10] Clomiphene acts as an antiestrogene and binds to estrogen receptors in hypothalamus and pituitary. This removes the contribution of estrogen (usually low levels in man), on the negative feedback resulting in increasing levels of GnRH, FSH, and LH. The dose of clomiphene is 12.5–50 mg daily. Serum testosterone, FSH, LH must be monitored and testosterone kept within normal. Therapy must be considered a failure if semen quality does not improve after 6 months.

Empirical therapy in patient with idiopathic infertility without the setting of hypogonadism with drug, such as GnRH, FSH, testosterone clomiphene, bromocriptine, and many vitamin supplements lack sound scientific basis.

Antioxidants such as vitamin E (400–1,200 IU per day) and glutathione (60 mg daily for 3–6 months)[10] may be useful in patients with proven elevated levels of semen reactive oxygen radicals. Kinin-enhancing drugs such as growth hormone are on clinical trials and may prove useful in improving spermatogenesis in oligospermic and azoospermic men with maturation arrest.[11]

■ REFERENCES

1. Murat Basar M, Atan A, Yildiz M, et al. Comparison of sertraline to fluoxetine with regard to their efficacy and side effects in the treatment of premature ejaculation. Arch Esp Urol. 1999;52:1008.
2. Althof SE. Prevalence, characteristics and implications of premature ejaculation/rapid ejaculation. J Urol. 2006;175:842.
3. Baldessarini RJ. Drug therapy for depression and anxiety. In: Brunton LL, Lazo JS, Parker KL (Eds). Goodman and Gilman's The pharmacological basis of therapeutics, 11th edn. McGraw-Hill, New-York, NY, 2006:429–59.
4. Montague DK, et al. AUA Erectile Dysfunction Guideline Update panel. AUA guideline on pharmacologic management of premature ejaculation. J Urol. 2004;172:290.
5. Broderick GA, Lue TF. Evaluation and management of erectile dysfunction and priapism. In: Walsh PC, Retik AB, Vaughan ED, Wein AJ (Eds.). Campbell's Urology, 8th edn. Saunders, Philadelphia, 2002:1619–72.
6. Bialecki ES, Bridges KR. Sildenafil relieves priapism in patients with sickle cell disease. Am J Med. 2002;113:252.
7. Burnett AL, Bivalacqua TJ, Champion HC, Musicki B. Feasibility of the use of phosphodiesterase type 5 inhibitors in a pharmacologic prevention program for recurrent priapism. J Sex Med. 2006;3:1077–84.
8. World Health Organization. WHO Manual for the standardized investigation and diagnosis of the infertile Couple. Cambridge University Press, Cambridge, UK, 2000.
9. World Health Organization. WHO laboratory manual for the examination of human semen and spermcervical mucus interaction, 4th edn. Cambridge University Press, Cambridge, UK, 1999.
10. Turek PJ. Male infertility. In: Tanagho EA, Mcttnninch TW (Eds.). Smith General Urology, 17th edn. McGraw-Hill, 2008; 684–726.
11. Ovesen P, Jorgensen JO, Kjaer T, et al. Growth hormone treatment of subfertile males. Fertil Steril. 1996;66:292–8.

SECTION 2

MEDICAL TREATMENT OF UROLOGICAL CANCER

Renal Cell Carcinoma
Ismaila A Mungadi, (Late) Hyacinth N Mbibu, Abdullahi Abdulwahab-Ahmed

Bladder Cancer
Ismaila A Mungadi, Mohamed H Kamel, Ngwobia P Agwu

Prostate Cancer
Ismaila A Mungadi, Olayiwola B Shittu, Abdullahi Abdulwahab-Ahmed

Testicular Cancer
Ismaila A Mungadi, Abdulkadir A Salako

Squamous Cell Carcinoma of the Penis
Ismaila A Mungadi, Abdullahi Abdulwahab-Ahmed

Nephroblastoma (Wilms' Tumor)
Christopher S Lukong, Emmanuel A Ameh

SECTION 2

MEDICAL TREATMENT OF UROLOGICAL CANCER

Renal Cell Carcinoma
Ismaila A Mungadi, (Late) Hyacinth N Mbibu, Abdullahi Abdulwahab-Ahmed

Bladder Cancer
Ismaila A Mungadi, Mohamed H Kamel, Ngwobia P Agwu

Prostate Cancer
Ismaila A Mungadi, Olayiwola B Shittu, Abdullahi Abdulwahab-Ahmed

Testicular Cancer
Ismaila A Mungadi, Abdulkadir A Salako

Squamous Cell Carcinoma of the Penis
Ismaila A Mungadi, Abdullahi Abdulwahab-Ahmed

Nephroblastoma (Wilms' Tumor)
Christopher S Lukong, Emmanuel A Ameh

CHAPTER 8

Renal Cell Carcinoma

Ismaila A Mungadi, (Late) Hyacinth N Mbibu, Abdullahi Abdulwahab-Ahmed

■ INTRODUCTION

Renal cell carcinoma (RCC) is an adenocarcinoma arising from renal tubular epithelium. It is the most fatal of all urologic malignancies. The incidence appears to be rising representing either a true rise or improved diagnosis of small renal masses. Genetic and environmental factors such as smoking have been implicated in the etiology of renal cell carcinoma. Genetic factors come into play in patients with Von Hippel-Lindau disease (VHLD), hereditary papillary renal cell carcinoma (HPRC), Birt Hogg-Dube disease (BHD) and hereditary leiomyomatosis and renal cell carcinoma (HLRCC).[1] Surgery is the mainstay of treatment of RCC. Systemic immunotherapy has an established role in patients with locally advanced and metastatic disease. Another attractive systemic therapy is the use of antiangiogenic agents. The role of these agents, however, as well as neoadjuvant immunotherapy, is being evaluated. The expected response of various modalities will depend on cell type as well as the stage of the disease. Renal cell carcinoma may be classified according to widely applied Robson's modification of Flock and Kadesky or the TNM system[2] (Table 8.1). Standardized staging is necessary to allow for evaluation of various prognostic and therapeutic models.

■ DRUG TREATMENT OF RCC

Renal cell carcinoma is resistant to conventional cytotoxic and hormonal therapy. The mainstay of systemic drug therapy at the moment is biological response modification in the form of immunotherapy. The role of angiogenic agents is currently being evaluated with encouraging results. Flow chart 8.1 shows an algorism of treatment of RCC.

Immunotherapy

Renal cell carcinoma is characterized by immunogenicity. There have been reported cases of spontaneous tumor resolution, dramatic shrinkage, prolonged disease stabilization, and positive response to immunotherapy.

Medical Treatment of Urological Cancer

Table 8.1: International TNM staging system for renal cell carcinoma, 2002

T: Primary Tumor	
TX	Primary tumor cannot be assessed
T0	No evidence of primary tumor
T1	Tumor 7 cm or less in greatest diameter, confined to the kidney
	T1a ≤ 4 cm
	T1a > 4 cm but ≤ 7 cm
T2	Tumor more than 7 cm in greatest diameter confined to the kidney
T3	Tumor extends into major veins or invades adrenal gland or perinephric tissues but not beyond Gerota's Fascia
T3a	Tumor invades adrenal gland or perinephric tissues
T3b	Tumor extends grossly into renal vein(s) or vena cava below diaphragm
T3c	Tumor grossly extends into vena cava above diaphragm
T4	Tumor invades beyond Gerota's fascia
N: Regional Lymph Nodes	
NX	Regional lymph nodes cannot be assessed
N0	No regional lymph node metastasis
N1	Metastasis in a single regional lymph node
N2	Metastasis in more than one regional lymph node
M: Distant Metastases	
MX	Distant metastasis cannot be assessed
M0	No distant metastasis
M1	Distant metastasis

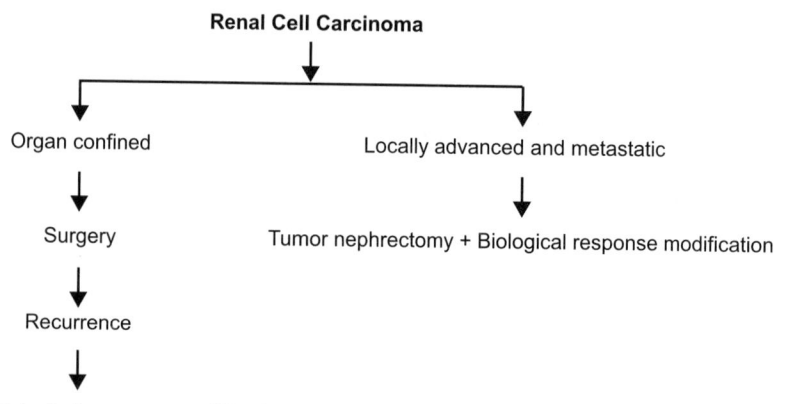

Flow chart 8.1: Suggested algorism for treatment of RCC

Altered T cell function and dendritic cell function have been reported in RCC.[3,4] Several immunomodulators show viable antitumor activity.[5] Cytokine immunomodulators showing antitumor activity in current use are Interferon L (INFL) and Interleukin-2 (IL-2). There is no difference clinically between

INFL2a and INF L2a and INF L2b4. The response rate to INFL is about 10–15% while that of IL-2 is about 15–20%. Patients with nonbulky tumors, clear cell histology, good performance status, and those who have had tumor nephrectomy are better responders to immunotherapy.

Antiangiogenic Agents

Renal cell carcinoma is a highly vascular tumor and depends heavily on angiogenesis for growth. Tumors must trigger angiogenesis under the control of cytokines and hormones to grow. Vascular endothelial growth factor (VEGF) and platelet-derived growth factor (PDGF) are proangiogenic factors, overexpressed in RCC, that can be targeted, and this inhibition has led to demonstrable clinical effect and disease stabilization.[6] Tyrosin kinase inhibitors (TKI) directed against VEGF receptor (VEGFR) and PDGFR such as sunitinib and sorafenib are approved in some countries. Thalidomide is also antiangiogenic and appears well tolerated in low doses. This is still under evaluation. VEGF can also be targeted using monocronal antibodies that bind to it. Bevacizumab is a recombinant humanized monoclonal antibody with such activity. It binds and neutralizes all the major forms of VEGF.[7]

Antiangiogenic agents appear promising and may open a new chapter in the drug therapy for RCC. These drugs may find a place not only in the treatment of systemic disease but also in neoadjuvant and multimodality therapies. However, more clinical studies are needed to determine these roles.

■ OUTLINE OF PHARMACOTHERAPY

Immunotherapy

Interferon Alpha

Mechanism of action: Interferons have antiviral and antitumor activity through several mechanisms. They induce protein kinase synthesis that selectively phosphorylate and inactivate proteins involved in protein synthesis. Interferons promote apoptosis, upregulate major histocompatibility complex (MHC), and tumor-associated antigens. They activate and enhance cytotoxic activity of macrophages, lymphocytes, and natural killer cells.

Properties: Interferons are inactivated if administered orally. Peak levels are achieved in 4–8 hours following intramuscular or subcutaneous injection. Conjugation of interferons to polyethylene glycol (PEG), called pegylations, prolongs absorption to allow weekly dosing.

Indications: Metastatic RCC in patients with good performance status.

Side effects: Influenza like synchrome, myelosuppression, granulocytopoiesis, thrombocytopenia, CNS including seizures, and depression, thyroiditis, hepatotoxicity, renal toxicity, autoimmunal diseases.

Contraindications: Consult product literature.

Interaction: Interferons may reduce the effects of various vaccines, increase the effects of aminophylline, and enhance the sedatives properties of opioids, antihistamines, and antidepressants. Also, consult product literature.

Dosage: Interferon L-2a (Roferon), Interferon L-2b (Intron A)—Consult manufacturers guide and relevant literature.

Preparation: Parenteral subcutaneous, IM or IV.

Interleukin 2

Mechanism of action: Interleukin 2 is a glycoprotein that induces and expands T cell response cytolytic for tumor cells. It also causes activation of natural killer cells and macrophages.

Properties: Must be given through continuous infusion due to its short half-life (13 minutes for IL-2L)

Indication: Metastatic renal cell carcinoma

Side effects: Inflammation and vascular leak due to expansion of cytotoxic lymphocytes, hypotension, arrhythmias renal damage, hepatotoxicity, gastrointestinal upset, confusion, fever, and myelodepression.

Contraindication/caution: See product literature.

Interaction: See product literature.

Dosage: Intercenkin—(IL-2, Aldeslenkin prolenkin)—has been administered at 600,000 units per kg IV every 8 hours for 5 days every other week for 2 cycles or 600,000 units per kg continuous IV for 5 days every other week for 2 cycles. Please see product literature for further guidance.

Antiangiogenic Agents

Monoclonal Antibody

Bevacizumab: This is a humanized monoclonal antibody against vascular endothelial Growth Factor. It has activity against clear cell renal cell carcinoma and is indicated in the treatment of metastatic RCC. If is formulated as a concentrate for intravenous infusion. Bevacizumab has potentially serious cardiovascular, gastrointestinal, hematological, allergic and nervous system side effects. For details please contact current pharmacotherapy literature and manufacturers' guide.

Tyrosin Kinase Inhibitors

Sunitinib, sorafenib: Protein kinases are critical signal transducing molecules. They transmit information to nucleus and influence gene transcription and DNA synthesis.[8] Tyrosine kinases have specific activity against tyrosine residues. Tyrosine kinases are abnormally expressed and activated in several tumors including RCC. Tyrosine kinase inhibitors have antitumor and antiangiogenic activity by targeting VEGF and PDGF receptors. These drugs are still being evaluated, and readers are advised to contact current pharmacotherapy literature and manufacturers' guide for further information.

REFERENCES

1. Vira MA, Novakovic KR, Pinto PA, Linehan WM, Genetic basis of kidney cancer: a model for developing molecular—targeted therapies. BJU Intl. 2007;99:1223-9.
2. Sabin LH, Wittekind CH (Eds.). International Union Against Cancer (IUCC). Classification of malignant diseases, 6th ed. Willy-Liss, New York, NY, 2002:193-5.
3. Troy AJ, Summers KL, Davidson PJ, Alkinson CH, Hart DN. Minimal recruitment and activation of dendritic cells within renal cell carcinoma. Clin Cancer Res. 1998;4:585-93.
4. Rayman P, Wesa AK, Richmond AL, et al. Effect of renal cell carcinoma on the development of type I T-Cell response. Clin Cancer Res. 2004;10:6360-5.
5. McDermott DF, Rni BI. Immunotherapy for metastatic renal cell carcinoma. BJU Intl. 2007;99:1282-8.
6. Srinivasan R, Amstrong AJ, Dhutt W, George DJ. Anti-angiogenetic therapy in renal cell cancer. BJU Intl. 2007;99:1296-1300.
7. Oosterwijk E, Divgi C, Bander NH. Active and passive immunotherapy: vaccines and antibodies. BJU Intl. 2007;99:1301-4.
8. Chabner BA, Amrein PC, Druker BJ, et al. Antineoplastic agents. In: Brunton LL, Lazo JS, Parker KL (Eds.). Goodman and Gilman's The pharmacological basis of therapeutics, 11th ed. McGraw-Hill, New York, NY. 2006:1315-1403.

CHAPTER 9
Bladder Cancer

Ismaila A Mungadi, Mohamed H Kamel, Ngwobia P Agwu

■ INTRODUCTION

Bladder cancer is the most common malignancy of the urinary tract. It is the second most common malignancy in men after prostate cancer.[1,2] It is three times more common in males than females.

Environmental carcinogens and genetic factors come into play in the etiology of bladder cancer. Alterations in *P53* and *Retinoblastoma* genes have been detected in some bladder cancer cases. Exposures to aromatic amines, cigarette smoking, infections, and chronic urethral irritation have all been implicated in the etiopathogenesis of bladder cancer. The commonest histological type of bladder cancer is transitional cell carcinoma (urothelial cancer) and arises from the urothelium. Other types include squamous cell carcinoma and adenocarcinoma. The squamous cell variety of bladder cancer is common in parts of Africa and Middle East, where urinary schistosomiasis is endemic and these usually present with muscle-invasive disease at the time of diagnosis, and is more resistant to chemotherapy; the only viable option for treatment is early radical cystectomy and urinary diversion.[3,4] The adenocarcinoma histological variety is rare, forms less than 2% of primary bladder cancers, and is usually found as a primary bladder lesion in urachal remnants, within intestinal urinary diversion or as metastasis from a primary focus of adenocarcinoma.[5]

There is a steady rise in incidence of bladder cancer and a corresponding fall in mortality from the disease since the 1950s. Bladder cancer and other urothelial malignancies tend to occur at multiple site and to re-occur. This is because the entire urothelium may be susceptible to malignancy due to "a field change." Therefore, drug treatment for bladder cancer is usually targeted at the urethelial variant and this may be beneficial not only for the treatment of late but also early disease.

Almost all patients with bladder cancers will present to the physician before their demise. A rational decision on the role of drugs in the management of bladder cancer can only be made after proper evaluation of patients, histologic typing, staging and grading of tumor. Table 9.1 shows the current TNM staging of bladder cancer.[6]

Table 9.1: TNM staging of bladder cancer

T-Primary Tumor	
TX	Primary tumor cannot be assessed
T0	No evidence of primary tumor
Ta	Non-invasive papillary carcinoma
Tis	Carcinoma in situ: "flat tumor"
T1	Tumor invades subepithelial connective tissue
T2	Tumor invades muscle
T2a	Tumor invades superficial muscle (inner half)
T2b	Tumor invades deep muscle (outer half)
T3	Tumor invades perivesical tissue
T3a	Microscopically
T3b	Macroscopically (extravesical mass)
T4	Tumor invades any of the following: prostate, uterus, vagina, pelvic wall, abdominal wall.
T4a	Tumor invades prostate, uterus or vagina
T4b	Tumor invades pelvic wall or abdominal wall
N- Lymph Nodes	
NX	Regional lymph nodes cannot be assessed
N0	No regional lymph node metastasis
N1	Metastasis in a single lymph node 2 cm or less in greatest dimension
N2	Metastasis in a single lymph node more than 2 cm but not more than 5 cm in greatest dimension
N3	Metastasis in a lymph node more than 5 cm in greatest dimension.
M – Distant Metastases	
MX	Distant metastasis cannot be assessed
M0	No distant metastasis
M1	Distant metastasis

Source: Sobin DH, Wittekind EH (Eds.). In: TNM classification of malignant tumors, 6th ed. Willy-Liss, New York, NY, 2002:199–202.

Grading of Urothelial Cancers

In 2004, WHO grading system for urothelial neoplasms classified these tumors into papillomas, papillary urothelial neoplasms of low malignant potential (PUNLMP), low-grade and high-grade urothelial carcinomas.[7,8]

Proper evaluation will enable the urologist to determine the extent of the disease and categorize the patients properly. The risk of progression and recurrence can also be estimated. The evaluation includes symptoms assessment, physical examination, ultrasonography, intravenous urography (IVU), computerized tomography scan (CT scan), urine cytology and cystoscopic examination, and biopsy and transurethral tumor resection. Fluorescene cystoscopy using photosensitizers such as 5-aminolevunic acid (5-ALA) and hexaminolevulinate (HAL) may improve tumor detection.

Treatment Options for Urethelial Cancer of the Bladder

The treatment options available in patients with urethelial bladder cancer are as follows:
1. Transurethral resection of bladder tumor (TURBT) intravesical immunotherapy
2. Intravesical chemotherapy
3. Cystectomy/lymphadenectomy
4. Radiotherapy
5. Systemic chemotherapy.

The choice of therapy depends on tumor stage, grade, cell type, accessibility, and clinical condition of the patient.

INTRAVESICAL THERAPY FOR SUPERFICIAL BLADDER CANCER

Superficial bladder cancer (SBC) refers to stage Ta, Tis, and T1 tumors of any grade. The risk of diseases' progression and recurrence determines justification for specific treatment in patients with SBC. Intravesical Bacille Calmette-Guérin (BCG) is the treatment of choice for primary carcinoma in situ (CIS) confined to the bladder. Response rate of 83–93% have been reported.[9,10]

Intravesical chemotherapy is also indicated to reduce progression, to prevent recurrence, and to remove subclinical area of tumor following transurethral extirpation of initial disease in patients with and T_1 lesion. Radical cystectomy (RC) is the treatment of choice in patients with T_1 tumors at high risk of recurrence and progression; these are patients with high-grade tumor, multifocal lesions coexisting CIS, and large lesions. Cystectomy is also indicated in patients with incomplete response and tumor recurrence.

INTRAVESICAL IMMUNOTHERAPY

Bacille Calmette-Guérin

Bladder tumor is an immunologically responsive tumor. This property coupled with intravesical accessibility has helped the establishment of standard therapy using BCG.[11] BCG may be used to treat Tis, residual Ta disease, and to prevent progression for high-risk patients and reduction of recurrence of superficial tumors. Intravesical administration of BCG promotes a local acute inflammatory and acute inflammatory granuloamatous reaction. Attachment of BCG to the urothelial cells including cancer cells triggers release of cytokines and chemokines resulting in recruitment of various types of immune cells into the bladder wall leading to stimulation of cell-mediated immunologic response that is predominantly T-helper/ inducer cell–mediated response.[12,13] BCG is very effective in the treatment of carcinoma in situ (CIS), and the initial response rate as high as 80% has been recorded.[14] Failure to respond to two 6-week courses or early recurrence is an indication for cystectomy. Patients with T_1 lesion and high-grade Ta lesion are also treated with BCG to prevent recurrence. Residual papillary tumors in patients not fit for resection may benefit from BCG treatment. Since its introduction in 1976 by Morales, intravesical BCG has played an important role in the management of high-grade nonmuscle invasive bladder cancer (NMIBC). Many studies have confirmed its value in reducing tumor recurrence following transurethral resection of bladder tumors (TURBT). Following endoscopic resection for high-grade (HG) Ta tumors followed by BCG the recurrence and progression rates are 47% and 25% respectively.[15] For HGT1 bladder cancer (tumor invasion of lamina propria), the recurrence and progression rates are 42% and 23%, respectively with a 14% delayed cystectomy rate.[16] In carcinoma in situ (CIS—flat, high-grade noninvasive cancer), the 5- and 10-year recurrence free rates are 63% and 54%. The 5- and 10-year progression free rates are 79% and 77% with 90% and 86% disease-specific survival at 5 and 10 years respectively.[17]

Following initial transurethral resection, patients with high-grade NMIBC are increasingly offered a second transurethral resection to eradicate residual tumor and confirm the tumor stage and grade. This is performed within 4 weeks of the initial diagnosis. Residual cancer is detected in up to 33% of patients.[18] Understaging of NMIBC at initial diagnosis, especially when no muscle is present in the specimen is a major problem. Understaging was observed in 78% of patients with clinical T1 tumors but muscularis propria was present in only 34%.[19] A recent report showed that a delay of more than 12 weeks from the time of transurethral resection to radical cystectomy significantly reduced the disease-free survival in muscle invasive bladder cancer.[20]

Bacille Calmette-Guérin is commonly given as a 6-week induction course, with an evaluation endoscopy 6 weeks later. If the patient has either a recurrent or new transitional cell carcinoma, the patient is often given the option of another 6-week course. Since BCG is perceived as the most effective adjunct to endoscopic tumor resection for CIS, HG Ta, andT1 bladder cancer,[21] and there is a paucity of options when this has failed, the definition of BCG failure is a most important one. Patients offered RC after failure of multiple courses of BCG have a much poorer prognosis.[22] Early RC and orthotopic urinary diversion in high-grade NMIBC cancer is associated with a reasonable quality of life.[23] Herr and Sogani[24] demonstrated that patients who have radical cystectomy offered less than 2 years from the start of BCG therapy had a better disease-pecific survival than if performed more than 2 years from the initiation of BCG. Table 9.2 identifies a variety of definitions for "BCG failure."

Table 9.2: Variety of definitions for "BCG failure"

Tumor Type	NCI [25]	EAU [26]	FICBT [27]	NCCN [28]
HG Ta/T1	Persistent T1 tumor despite 6 weeks course of BCG	T2 or higher HG NMIBC at both 3 and 6 months (2 courses of BCG) Worsening disease as increase stage, grade, higher number of recurrences or CIS	*BCG refractory*: Increase in tumor stage, grade or disease extent at 3 months. Failure to achieve a disease free state after 6 months of BCG treatment (either due to persistent or rapidly recurring disease) *BCG resistant*: Recurrence or persistence of disease at 3 months after the induction cycle. It is of lesser degree, stage, or grade, and is no longer present at 6 months from BCG retreatment with or without TUR *BCG relapsing*: Tumor recurs after 6 months of BCG (early <12 m, intermediate 12–24 m and late > 24 m) *BCG Intolerant*: Tumor recurs after less than an adequate course of therapy due to a BCG related adverse event	Persistence of cTa, cT1 no more than 2 cycles of 6 weeks of BCG
Bladder CIS	Persistent CIS despite 2 BCG courses	Persistent CIS despite 2 BCG courses	Persistent CIS despite 2 BCG courses	Persistent CIS despite 2 BCG courses
Prostatic Urethra CIS	NA	NA	Only in CIS confined to urothelium. Failure if CIS persists despite one 6 weeks course of BCG	In CIS confined to urothelium, failure if CIS persists despite 1 course. BCG and TURP may be tried only one time in tumor involving prostatic ductal acini

Note: NCI: National Cancer Institute, EAU: European Urological Association' FICBT: The First International Consultation on Bladder Tumors, NCCN: National Comprehensive Cancer Network

Interferon-Alpha

Difficulties in obtaining interferon and easy accessibility of BCG has reduced the usefulness of this drug in the management of superficial bladder cancers.

Keyhole Limpet Hemocyanin (KLH)

This is an immunogenic protein produced by a molusc, *Megathura crenulata*. KLH has been shown to be more effective than mitomycin $C^{29,30}$ and is at least as effective as BCG. Unavailability also, limits its usefulness in the management of SBC.

■ INTRAVESICAL CHEMOTHERAPY

The most commonly used agents are adriamycin, epirubicin, and mitomycin C. The use of thiotepa is limited by toxicity. Thiotepa, being a low-molecular weight drug, is readily absorbed leading to bone marrow depression. Other second-line drugs used in SBC are valrubicin and mitoxantrone. Mitoxantrone requires fewer installations and is as effective of mitomycin C or epirubicin at half the number of installations.

■ PHOTODYNAMIC THERAPY

This involves use of photosensitizing agents, which when activated by light produce cancer cell death. If systemically administered (e.g. porphyrins), patients must wait for 3 days to allow the substance to clear from normal tissue before intravesical red laser treatment is given. The skin is also photosensitized and the patient must stay out of sunlight for several weeks. The problem of systemic photosensitizers (photofrin) has led to the development of intravesical photosensitizers such as 5-aminolevulenic acid (ALA), which is actively taken up by urothelium and is rapidly metabolized.[31,32] Photodynamic therapy is still undergoing evaluation.

■ COMBINATION THERAPY AND TIMING

Bacille Calmette-Guérin or chometherapeutic agent is usually given as a single agent. Combinations such as BCG and mitomycin C or mitomycin C and adriamycin do not appear to offer special advantage. BCG is administered after a two-week delay from tumor resection to reduce side effects. Mitomycin C, epirubicin or adriamycin can be administered within 6 hours of resection. This early instillation therapy reduces recurrence rate without significantly increasing side effect.[33]

■ INVASIVE BLADDER CANCER

Advanced bladder cancer comprises of three distinctive entities; inoperable disease due to local extension, grossly involved pelvic or para-aortic nodes, metastatic disease at presentation or recurrence after radical cystectomy. Drug treatment in these patients could be adjuvant or as neoadjuvant therapy.[34]

Neoadjuvant

The gold standard treatment of invasive bladder cancer is radical cystectomy and urinary diversion, but many patients present later with metastatic disease. Chemotherapy given before cystectomy is referred to as neoadjuvant therapy.

Neoadjuvant chemotherapy is given with the hope of achieving the following benefits.
- Downstaging tumors thus converting an inoperable tumor to operable disease.
- Attacking micrometastasis at an early stage.
- The sensitivity of tumor to chemotherapeutic agent is tested in vivo, thus allowing for the continuation of the neoadjuvant regimen postoperatively.
- Chemotherapy may be better tolerated before cystectomy.

Cisplatin-based neoadjuvant combination has been an established standard in patients with muscle invasive bladder cancer and has demonstrated improved overall survival.[35,36] Despite these presumed advantages, only a modest 5–70% increased survival has been demonstrated.[37,38] Also neoadjuvant therapy has a potential disadvantage of delaying surgery.

Adjuvant

There is no evidence that systemic therapy after cystectomy offers survival advantage in patents with T_1–T_2 disease. The role of adjuvant therapy in patients with T_3/T_4 and/or N+ is under debate.[39,40]

■ SYSTEMIC CHEMOTHERAPY FOR METASTATIC DISEASE

Patients with metastatic bladder cancer should be treated with chemotherapy. Cisplatin-based combination chemotherapy has long been the preferred regimen.[41] Complete response rate of 20% is expected with cisplatin, methotrexate, and vinblastine (CMV) and methotrexate, vinblastine, doxorubicin, and cisplatin (MVAC) regimens.[42,43] However, some patients experience high rate of toxicity thus necessitating newer drug combinations. A combination of cisplatin/carboplatin and newer agents such as gemcitabine, paclitaxel, or docetaxel may give response rate ranging from 25% to 83%.[44–46]

Carboplatin-based combination chemotherapy has been found useful in patients with impaired renal function; although, it is not as effective as cisplatin-based combination. In addition to these chemotherapeutic drugs, patients with metastatic bladder cancer require adjunctive and palliative care including use of bisphosphonates that do not act to ensure skeletal integrity but have been recently found to have anticancer effects.[47,48]

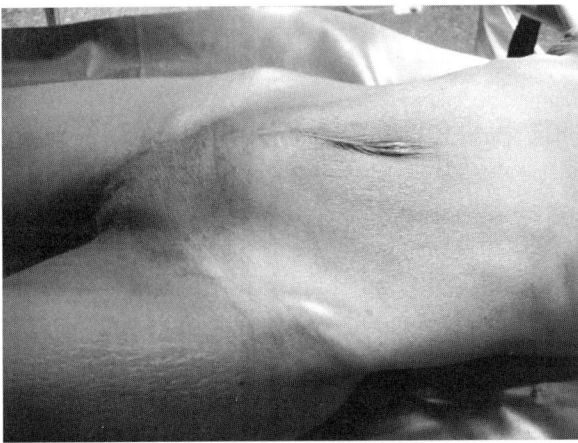

Fig. 9.1: A lady with advanced bladder carcinoma
(*For color version, see plate 2*)

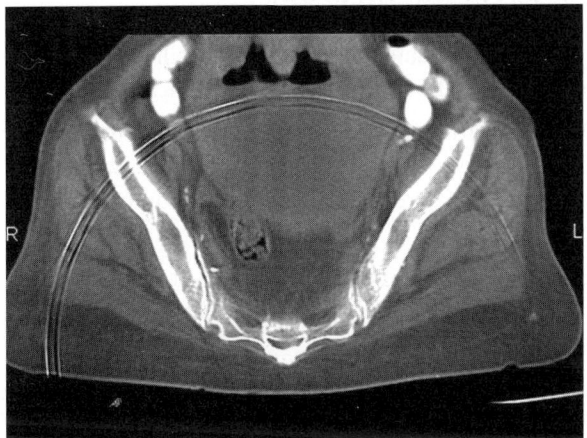

Fig. 9.2: Computerized tomographic scan showing tumor mass almost obliterating the bladder lumen

Figures 9.1 and 9.2 show a lady with advanced bladder carcinoma.

OTHER GUIDELINES

Drug Combination

Combination therapy is superior to single agent regimens.[49-51] Also, it appears that cisplatin-based combinations are superior to other combination without cisplatin.[52] Various drug combinations are shown in Table 9.3.

Variant Histology

The response rates described earlier are all based on transitional cell–type carcinoma. Patients with mixed histology are expected to respond favorably.

Table 9.3: Cytotoxic drug combinations for bladder cancer

Cisplatin, methotrexate, vinblastine (CMV)
Methotrexate, vinblastine, adriamycin, cisplatin (MVAC)
Gemcitabine and cisplatin (carboplatin or Gemcitabine, paclitaxel (or Docetaxel).
Gemcitabine, Paclitaxel (or Docetaxel and cisplatin (or carboplatin)
Cisplatin (or carboplatin) and paclitaxel (or docetaxel).

Other cell types may respond differently. The optimal drug choice and combination for adenocarcinoma, small cell carcinoma, and squamous cell carcinoma has yet to be determined.

DETAILS OF PHARMACOTHERAPY FOR BLADDER CANCER[14, 33, 43–46, 49–51, 53–56]

Bacillus Calmette-Guérin (BCG)

Properties: BCG is an attenuated live culture of bacillus of Calmette and Guérin strain at mycobacterium bovis. Its mechanism of action is unclear.

Indication: As the sole treatment in carcinoma in situ; initial response expected in 70–80% of patients. It is also indicated in patients with residual papillary tumor and to prevent recurrence following resection of Tl and high-grade Ta tumors.

Side effects: Fever, chills, malaise, urinary frequency, dysuria, cystitis hypersensitivity, shock, granulomatous prostatitis, and systemic BCG infection.

Contraindication: Active tuberculosis, UTI, HIV infection, impaired immune response, pyrexia of undetermined origin, hematuria, breastfeeding and pregnancy, unhealed urethral, and bladder injuries.

Caution: History of tuberculosis, traumatic catheterization (delay until healed).

Dose/Administration: 10 million organisms per instillation, reconstituted with 50 ml saline administered soon after reconstitution and not less than 2 weeks after resection. Administered under gravity and retained for 2 hours. A 6-weekly course is given as induction. Alternative treatment must be considered if patient does not respond after 2 courses. Maintenance treatment may be given using 2 to 3 additional top-up doses at 3–6 months intervals.

Preparation: Freeze-dried powder of attenuated mycobecteriun boris, Connoausht Spain (Immucyst) TICE Spain (OncoTICE).

Mitomycin C

Properties: Mitomycin C is an antibiotic derived from *Streptococcus caespitosus*. It contains a quinolone and azauridine groups. The quinolone group undergoes intracellular chemical reduction, with subsequent release of methoxy group. By this, DNA synthesis and cross-linkage of DNA at specific positions are inhibited.

Indication: Direct instillation for the treatment of superficial bladder cancer, systemic absorption is limited due to large molecular weight at 334 kD.

Side effects: Chemical cystitis, skin rashes, nausea and myelodepression, lung fibrosis, renal damage, and rarely bladder fibrosis.

Contraindication: Lactation, pregnancy.

Dose and administration: 20–60 mg in 20 mL–40 mL saline weekly for 6 to 8 weeks retained for 2 hours may be administered as a single dose immediate post resection to reduce to recurrence.

Preparation: Injection, powder.

Doxorubicin

Properties: Doxorubicin is an anthracycline cytotoxic antibiotic. It is isolated from Streptococcus. Doxorubicin either interacts directly with DNA or forms complexes with the ATP-dependent topoisomerase enzyme. This enzyme plays a major role in DNA replication and repair by realignment of breakages and fragments of DNA. As such formation of the doxorubicin-topoisomerase II–DNA complex inhibits re-ligation of broken DNA resulting in apoptosis. Doxorubicin also has the propensity to react with iron to form free radicals. This is as a result of the presence of quinine and hydroquinone moieties on adjacent rings that enhance the loss or gain of electrons. These free radicals form reactive intermediates that disrupt nucleic acid bases.

Doxorubicin is given intravenously. It is metabolized in the liver with significant rapid uptake of the drug by the heart, kidney, lungs, and spleen. It, however, does not cross the blood-brain barrier. It is excreted as inactive products, mainly in the biliary tracts.

Indication: Intravesical therapy, combination therapy for bladder cancer.

Side effects: Doxorubicin causes cumulative cardiomyopathy with potentially fatal heart failure, dose-limiting myelosuppression, nausea, vomiting, anorexia, anemia, stomatitis, and alopecia. It also produces severe local tissue toxicity.

Indication: It is useful in several solid tumors including transitional cell carcinoma (TCC) of the bladder.

Precaution: Drug should be handled with care because it causes tissue irritation. Severe tissue necrosis results from extravasations of the drug. Doses should be reduced in patients with hepatic impairments.

Contraindication: Lactation and pregnancy.

Drug interaction: There is an increased risk of toxicity when used concomitantly with clozapin and cyclosporine. It reduces absorption of phenytoin and digoxin. Doxorubicin appears to inhibit the effect of stavudine.

Dosage: It is given at a dose of 50–70 mg per square meter rapid IV infusion and repeated every 21 days.

Preparation: Doxorubicin hydrochloride injection.

Epirubicin

Epirubicin is an anthracycline cytotoxic antibiotic and structurally related to doxorubicin. Its metabolism, mechanism of action and antineoplastic activity are generally similar to doxorubicin.

It is used for the treatment and prophylaxis of superficial bladder tumors by direct instillation.

Methotrexate

Properties: Methotrexate is an antimetabolite used to treat a variety of malignancies. Methotrexate inhibits the enzyme dihydrofolate reductase. This enzyme converts folic acid to a series of dihydrofolate cofactors in a one carbon transfer reaction that is crucial in the de novo synthesis of precursors of DNA (purines and pyrimidines).

Methotrexate is readily absorbed from the gastrointestinal tract. Distribution of the drug into body spaces such as pleural and peritoneal cavity is slow. About 50% of methotrexate is bound to plasma protein and up to 90% of a given dose is excreted unchanged in urine within 48 hours, and a small amount is excreted in stool.

Indication: Combination therapy for bladder cancer.

Side effects: Primary toxicity of methotrexate is its effect on bone marrow and intestinal epithelium with risk of spontaneous hemorrhage and infection and myelosuppression in patients with impaired renal function. Others are mucositis, alopecia, dermatitis, nephrotoxicity, abortion, defective oogenesis and spermatogenesis, teratogenesis, interstitial pneumonitis, and hepatic fibrosis.

Precaution: Methotrexate is given orally, IV, IM, or intrathecally. It should be avoided in patients with significant pleural effusion and ascites because it accumulates in these fluids, serving as a site for storage and slow release of drug with resultant high plasma concentrations and more severe toxic effects. It should be used with caution in hepatic and renal impairments.

Contraindications: Pregnancy, breastfeeding.

Drug interactions: The antifolate effect of methotrexate is increased by concomitant use of nitrous oxide. NSAIDs, ciprofloxacin, and penicillin reduce its excretion, thereby increasing risk of toxicity. Absorption of methotrexate is reduced by neomycin and phenytoin. Sulfamethaxazole, doxycycline, trimethoprim, and corticosteroids interact with methotrexate to increase its hematological toxicities.

Dosage: See manufacturers' guide and published protocols.

Preparation: Oral, IM, IV.

Leucovorin Calcium (Folinic Acid)

It is also called folinic acid and represents the 5-formyl derivative of tetrahydrofolic acid. Folinic acid is used to prevent the toxic effect of the folate antagonist, for example, methotrexate, especially their high dose-induced toxic effect and to enhance recovery from myelosuppression and mucositis. This is referred to as "folinic acid rescue" used in case of folic acid deficiency. Folinic acid should not be used concomitantly with methotrexate. It is given either IM, IV, or IV infusion. Started 24 hours after the commencement of methotrexate. It is given as 15 mg and repeated every 6 hours for 24 hours. Subsequent doses could be given orally to prevent methotrexate-induced adverse effects.

It is contraindicated in lactating and pregnant mothers. Adverse effects include fever and hypersensitivity reaction.

Cisplatin

Properties: Cisplatin (cis-diaminedichloroplatinum II) is a divalent water-soluble, platinum–containing compound. Cisplatin enters cells by diffusion and by an active cu^{2+} transporter. Inside the cells, it reacts with nucleophilic sites on DNA and proteins. Cisplatin is given intravenously only. It has an initial plasma elimination half-life of 25–50% minutes following IV administration. More than 90% of the drug is bound covalently to plasma proteins. High concentrations are found in tissues of the kidney, liver, intestine, and testes. The drug has poor CNS penetration. It is predominantly excreted by the kidney with minimal intestinal and biliary excretion.

Indication: It is used alone or in combination for treatment of testicular, and bladder cancer

Side effects: Treatment with cisplatin may be complicated by severe nausea and vomiting. It also causes nephrotoxicity, ototoxicity peripheral neuropathy, myelosuppression, and hypomagnesemia.

Precaution: To prevent renal toxicity, it is important to establish a chloride diuresis by the infusion of 1–2 liters of normal saline prior to treatment. It is important not to use needles or aluminum-containing equipment when preparing or administering cisplatin because aluminum reacts with and inactivates cisplatin.

Contraindication: Pregnancy and breastfeeding.

Drug interaction: There is increased risk of primary toxicity when cisplatin is given with bleomycine and methotrexate. Risk of nephrotoxicity and of ototoxicity is increased when given along with aminoglycosides, vancomycin, and diuretics.

Dosage: It is 20 mg per square meter a day for 5 days, 20–30 mg weekly for 3–4 weeks or 100 mg per square meter given once every 4 weeks. Appropriate amounts of cisplatin are diluted in solution of dextrose or saline and administered IV over 4 hours. Also, see published protocols.

Carboplatin

Properties: Carboplatin is a water-soluble platinum–containing compound. Though significantly different from cisplatin in metabolism and toxicological properties, carboplatin shares similar mechanism of action and chemical spectrum with cisplatin.

Carboplatin is administered intravenously, it is less reactive than cisplatin with significant amount unbound to plasma proteins. It has a half-life of 2 hours and is excreted by the kidneys.

Indications: Carboplatin is an effective alternative to cisplatin for responsive tumors in patients with impaired renal function and intolerable cisplatin toxicities.

Side effects: Carboplatin causes more myelosuppression than cisplatin; however, it causes less severe nausea, vomiting, neurotoxicity, nephrotoxicity, and ototoxicity. Late effects are leukopenia, thrombocytopenia, and hepatic dysfunction.

Precaution: Although carboplatin is generally more tolerated with fewer toxicity, dose reduction may be required in patients with impaired renal function.

Contraindication: Pregnancy and lactation.

Drug interactions: There is increased risk of ototoxicity and nephrotoxicity when used concomitantly with aminoglycosides, vancomycin, capreomycin, clozapin, and diuretics. It reduces absorption of digoxin and phenytoin.

Dose: Carboplatin is given at 360 mg per square meter IV every 4 weeks

Preparation: IV.

Vincristine

Properties: Vincristine is a vinca alkaloid antimitotic agent. Vincristine is a cell-cycle specific agent that inhibits cellular mitosis. It binds specifically to β-tubulin and blocks its ability to polymerize with α-tubulin into microtubules with resultant absence of mitotic spindle, as such duplicated chromosomes cannot align along the division plate leading to arrest of mitosis at metaphase.

It is extensively metabolized in the liver and the conjugates and metabolites are excreted in bile with a small fraction of the dose excreted in urine uncharged. In patients with hepatic dysfunction (bilirubin ≤ 3 mg per day) a 75% reduction in dose is advisable. It has the expected advantage of slower elimination and greater tissues distribution when compared to the unmodified drug. It has an elimination half-life of 1–20 hours.

Indication: Metastatic bladder and testicular cancers.

Side effects: The clinical manifestation of the toxicity of vincristine is neurotoxicity. It may cause numbness and tingling sensation of the extremities, severe constipation, reversible alopecia, myelosuppression, and loss of deep tendon reflexes.

Precaution: Vincristine sulfate comes in powder preparations of 1 mg or 5 mg vial made into solution for intravenous use only. Extravasations during intravenous administration of vincristine should be avoided because this leads to severe pain and necrosis of surrounding tissues. Inadvertent intrathecal vincristine administration produces devastating and fatal central neurotoxicity with seizures and irreversible coma.

Contraindication: Breastfeeding and pregnant mothers.

Drug interaction: Metabolism of vincristine is inhibited by antifungal agents such as itraconazole with increased risk of neurotoxicity. It should not be used concomitantly with antipsychotic, for example clozapine (agranulocytosis). Metabolism of vincristine is inhibited by calcium channel blocker such as nifedipine.

Dosage: See manufacturers' guide and published protocols.

Preparation: IV.

Gemcitabine

Properties: Gemcitabine is a difluoro analog of deoxycytidine. It is actively taken into the intracellular compartment with the help of nucleoside transporters. Here it undergoes phosphorylation by deoxycytidine kinase to produce the triphosphate nucleoside that in turn inhibit DNA synthesis.

The drug is given by intravenous infusion. It is metabolized in the liver and has a short half-life of about 15 minutes. Gemcitabine is eliminated in urine in its inactive form; however, clearance varies among individuals, slower in women and elderly and is dose-dependent.

Indications: It is used in combination therapy for treatment of advanced bladder cancer.

Side effects: The most significant toxicity of gemcitabine is myelosuppression. This is related to the duration of infusion. Others are elevated liver transaminasis, asthenia, intestinal pneumonitis, and flu-like syndrome. Hemolytic ureamic syndrome has been reported.

Precaution: Gemcitabine should be used with care in patients with hepatic and renal impairment.

Contraindication: Lactation and pregnancy.

Dosage: 1–1.2 g per square meter over 30 minutes on days 1, 8, and 15 of each 28-day cycle.

Preparation: IV.

Paclitaxel and Docetaxel

Properties: Paclitaxel is an alkaloid ester, and the first compound in the group; it was isolated from the bark of the Western yew tree. A side chain attached to the taxane ring is essential for its cytotoxicity. The related semisynthetic, more potent analog docetaxel results from modification of this side chain. Docetaxel shares similar range of pharmacological activity with paclitaxel but is less toxic. This is because unlike paclitaxel, it is more soluble. Paclitaxel binds selectively to the β subunit of microtubules resulting in enhancement of tubulin polymerization and promotion of assembly of microtubules and aberrant structures derived from microtubules. This causes arrest of mitosis. Paclitaxel is metabolized by the liver, with a half-life of 10–14 hours and excreted unchanged in the urine. Docetaxel's half-life is about 12 hours, and also undergoes hydroxylation by hepatic metabolism and production of inactive products.

Indications: The taxanes are used in various combinations for the treatment of metastatic bladder, prostate, and testicular cancers.

Side effects: Paclitaxel causes severe hypersensitivity reaction, myelosuppresion, peripheral neuropathy, arrhythmias, alopecia, muscle pain, nausea, and vomiting. Docetaxel may cause persistent fluid retention during treatment. Oral dexamethasone is given to relieve edema and hypersensitivity reactions.

Precaution: Premedication with H2-receptor blockers, antihistamines and corticosteroid is required to prevent the severe hypersensitivity reactions of paclitaxel; however, this may rarely occur despite premedication. Because of its poor solubility, paclitaxel must be administered in a vehicle of 50% ethanol and 50% polyethoxylated castor oil.

Drug interaction: Paclitaxel reduces absorption of phenytoin. There is a risk of agranulocytosis when used concomitantly with clozapine. Plasma concentrations of paclitaxel are increased by nelfinavir and ritonavir. Studies have shown drug interactions between docetaxel and erythromycin, ketoconazole and cyclosporin.

Contraindication: Pregnancy and lactation.
Dosage: See manufacturers' guide and published protocols.

REFERENCES

1. Greenlee RT, Murray T, Bolden S, Wings PA. Cancer statistics, 2000. CA Cancer J Clin. 2000;50:7.
2. Feldman AR, Kessler L, Myers MH, Naughton MD. The Prevalence of cancer: estimates based on the Connecticut Tumor Registry. N Engl J Med. 1986;315:1394.
3. Botelho MC, Machado JC, Correia da Costa JM. Schistosoma haematobium and bladder cancer: What lies beneath? Virulence. 2010;1:84–7.
4. Izzo L, Pietrasanta D, Izzo P, Caputo M, Di Cello P, Meloni P, Bolognese A. A case of relapsing secondary bladder adenocarcinoma after right colonic cancer. Nat Clin Pract Urol. 2008;5:403–7.
5. Stenzl A, Witjes JA, Cowan NC, Santis MD, Kuczyk M, Lebret T, Merseburger AS. EUA Guidelines on Bladder Cancer; Muscle-invasiveand Metastatic 2011.
6. Sobin DH, Wittekind EH (Eds.). In: TNM classification of malignant tumors, 6th ed. Willy-liss, New York, NY, 2002:199–202.
7. Kirkali Z, Cham T, Manoharan M, et al. Bladder cancer: epidemiology, staging and grading and diagnosis. Urology. 2005;66(Supp; 6A):4–34.
8. Askeland EJ, Newton MR, O'Donnell MA, Luo Y. Bladder cancer Immunotherapy: BCG and beyond. Advances in Urology 2012, Article ID 181987. 13 pages.
9. Lamm DL, Blumenstein BA, Crissman JD, et al. Maintainance Bacillus Calmette-Guérin immunotherapy for recurrent Ta T1 and carcinoma-in situ transistional cell carcinoma of the bladder; a randomized South-west Oncology Group study. J Urol. 2000;163:1124.
10. Brusman SA. Experience with bacillus Calmette-Guérin in patients with superficial bladder cancer. J Urol. 1982;128:27.
11. Morales A, Nickel JC, Wilson JWL. Dose response of bacillus Calmette-Guérin in the treatment of superficial bladder cancer. J Urol. 1992;157:1256–8.
12. Kapoor R, Vijjan V, Singh P. Bacillus Calmette-Guérin in management of superficial bladder cancer. Indian J Urol. 2008;24:72–6.
13. Pliarchopoulou K, Laschos K, Pectasides D. Current chemotherapeutic options for the treatment of advanced bladder cancer: A Review. Urologic Oncology: Seminars and Original Investigations, 2013;31:281–392.
14. Brosman SA. Experience with bacillus Calmette-Guérin in patients with superficial bladder carcinoma. J Urol. 1982;128:27–30.
15. Lebret T, Bohin D, Kassardjian Z, et al. Recurrence, progression and success in stage Ta grade 3 bladder tumors treated with low-dose bacillus Calmette-Guérin insillations. J Urol. 2000;163:63.
16. Peyromaure M, Guerin F, Amsellem- Ouazana D, et al. Intravesical bacillus Calmette-Guérin therapy for stage T1 grade 3 transitional cell carcinoma of the bladder: recurrence, progression and survival in a study of 57 patients. J Urol. 2003;169:2110.

17. Gofrit ON, Pode D, Pizov G, Zorn KC, Katz R, Duvdevani M, Shapiro A. The natural history of bladder carcinoma in-situ after initial response to bacillus Calmette-Guérin immunotherapy. Urol Oncol. 2009;27:258.
18. Divrik T, Yildirim U, Eroglu AS, et al. Is a second transurethral resection necessary for newly diagnosed pT1 bladder cancer? J Urol. 2006;175:1258.
19. Cheng L, Neumann RM, Weaver AL, et al. Grading and staging of bladder carcinoma in transurethral resection specimens. Am J Clin Pathol. 2000;113:275-9.
20. Gore JL, Lai J, Setodji CM, Litwin MS, Saigal CS. Urologic diseases in America. America Project. Mortality increases when radical cystectomy is delayed more than 12 weeks: results from a surveillance, epidemiology and end results medicare analysis. Cancer. 2009;115:988-96.
21. Herr HW, Morales A. History of bacillus Calmette-Guérin and bladder cancer: an immunotherapy success story. J Urol. 2008 Jan;179(1):53-6.
22. Lambert EH, Pierorazi PM, Olsson CA, Benson MC, McKiernan JM, Poon S. The increasing use of intavesical therapies for stage T1 bladder cancer coincides with decreasing survival after cystectomy. BJU Intl. 2007;100:33-6.
23. Esrig D, Freeman JA, Stein JP, Skinner DG. Early cystectomy for clinical stage T1 transitional cell carcinoma of the bladder. Semin Urol Oncol. 1997;15:154-60.
24. Herr HW, Sogani PC. Does early cystectomy improve the survival of patients with high risk superficial bladder tumors? J Urol. 2001;166:1296-9.
25. http://www.cancer.gov/cancertopics/pdq/treatment/bladder/Health Professional/page7. Access date 26 May, 2009.
26. http://www.uroweb.org/fileadmin/tx_eauguidelines/2009/Full/TaT1_BC.pdf. Access date May 15, 2009.
27. Neider AM, Brausi M, Lamm D, et al. T1 Urothelial carcinoma of the Bladder, In: Soloway M, Carmac A (Eds.). Bladder tumors. Health Publications Ltd, Paris, 2006:191-217.
28. http://www.nccn.org/professionals/physician gls/PDF?bladder.pdf.Access date May 26, 2009.
29. Olssson C, Chute R, Rao C. Immunologic reduction of bladder cancer recurrence rate. J Urol. 1979;111:173.
30. Jurinic CD, Engelmann V, Gasch J, et al. Immunotherapy in bladder cancer with keyhole limpet haemocyanin: a randomized study. J Urol. 1988;139:723.
31. Kriegmain M, Stepp H, Streaubach P, et al. Fluorescence cystoscopy following intravesical instillationof 5- aminolevenulinic acid: a new procedure with high sensitivity if highly visible urothelial neoplasms. Urol Intl. 1995;55:190.
32. Walther MM, Delancy TF, Smith PD, et al. Phase 1 trial of photoluminescence therapy in the treatment of recurrent superficial transitional cell carcinoma of the bladder. Urology. 1997;50:199.
33. Malkowicz SB. Management of superficial bladder cancer. In: Walsh PC, Retik AB, Vaughan ED, Wein AJ (Eds.). Campbell's urology, 8th ed. Saunders, Philaldelphia, 2002:2785-2802.
34. Meeks JJ, Bellmunt J, Bochner BH, et al. A systematic review of neoadjuvant and adjuvant chemotherapy of muscle invasive bladder cancer. Eur Urol. 2012;62:523-33.

35. Elderfrawy A, Soloway MS, Katkoori D, Singal R, Pam D, Manoharan M. Neoadjuvant and adjuvant chemotherapy for muscle invasive bladder cancer: The likelihood of initiation and completion. Indian J Urol. 2012;28:424–6.
36. Fletcher A, Choudhury A, Alam N. Metastatic bladder cancer: a review of current management. ISRN Urology. 2011; Article ID 545241.
37. Advanced bladder cancer meta-analysis collaboration, neoadjuvant chemotherapy in invasive bladder cancer; a systematic review and meta-analysis. Lancet. 2003:361(9373):1927–34.
38. Winquist E, Kirchner TS, Segal R, Chin J, Lukka H. Genitourinary cancer diseases site group, cancer care Ontario programme in evidence-based care practice guidelines initiative, neoadjuvant chemotherapy for transitional cell carcinoma of the bladder: a systematic review and meta-analysis. J Urol. 2004;171(2Pt 1):651–569.
39. Cohen SM, Goel A, Phillips J, Ennis RD, Grossbard ML. The role if perioperative chemotherapy in the treatment of urothelial cancer. Oncologist. 2006;11(6):630–40.
40. Sylvester R. Sternberg C. The role of adjuvant combination chemotherapy after cystectomy in locally advanced bladder cancer: what we do not know \and why. Ann Oncol. 2000;11(7):851–6.
41. Nicholson S. Chemotherapy of bladder cancer in patients with impaired renal function. Nat Rev Urol. 2012;9:52–7.
42. Harker WG, Freiha FS, Palmer JM, et al. Cisplatin, methotrexate, and vinblastine (CMV): an effective chemotherapy regimen for metastatic transitional cell carcinoma of the urinary tract. A Northern California Oncology Group study. J Clin Oncol. 1985;3:1463–70.
43. Stockle M, Wellek S, Voges G, et al. Advanced bladder cancer (stages pT3b, pT4a, pN1 and pN2): Improved survival after radical cystectomy and 3 adjuvant cycles of chemotherapy. Results of a controlled prospective study. J Urol. 1992;148:302–6.
44. Pycha A, Posch B, Schnack B, et al. Paclitaxel and carboplatin in patients with metastatic transitional cell cancer of the urinary tract. Urology. 1999;53:510–5.
45. Zielinski CC, Grbovic M, Brodowicz T, et al. Paclitaxel and carboplatin in patients with metastatic urothelial cancer: results of a phase II trial. Br J Cancer. 1998;78:370–4.
46. Sengelov L, Lund B, Engelholm SA. Docetaxel and cisplatin in metastatic urothelial cancer: A phase II study. J Clin Oncol. 1998;16:3392–7.
47. Koul HK, Koul S, Meacham RB. New role for an established drug? Bisphosphonates as potential anti-cancer agents. Prostate Cancer Prostatic Dis. 2012;15:111–9.
48. Fitzpatrick JM, Colombel M, Saad F, Sternberg CN, Tubaro A. Treatment strategies in advanced Cancer/ Genitourinary Malignancies: the use of Bisphosphonates across the continuum. Eur Urol. 2009;Suppl 8:733–7.
49. Soloway MS, Einstein A, Corder MP, et al. A comparison of cisplatin and the combination of cisplatin and cyclophosphamide in advanced urothelial cancer. A National Bladder Cancer Collaborative Group A study. Cancer. 1983;52(5):767–72.

50. Troner M, Birch R, Omura GA, et al. Phase III comparison of cisplatin alone versus cisplatin, doxorubicin and cyclophosphamide in the treatment of bladder (urothelia) cancer: a Southeastern Cancer study Group trial. J Urol. 1987;137(4):660–2.
51. Khandekar JD, Elson PJ, DeWys WD, et al. Comparative activity and toxicity of cis-diamminedichloroplatinum (DDP) and a combination of doxorubicin, cyclophosphamide, and DDP in disseminated transitional cell carcinomas of the urinary tract. J Clin Oncol. 1985;3(4):539–45.
52. Mead GM, Russell M, Clark P, et al. A randomised trial comparing methotrexate and vinblastine (MV) with cisplatine, methotrexate and vinblastine (CMV) in advanced transitional cell carcinoma: results and report on prognostic factors in Medical Research Council study. MRC Advanced Bladder Cancer Working Party. Br J Cancer. 1998;78:1067–75.
53. Chabner BA, Amrein PC, Michaelson MD, et al. Chemotherapy of neoplastic diseases. In: Brunton LL, Lazo JS, Parker KL (Eds.). Goodman and Gilman's The pharmacological basis of therapeutics, 11th ed. McGraw-Hill, New-York, NY, 2006:1315–1404.
54. British National Formulary. BMJ and RPS, London, 2008;56:453–96.
55. Whelan P. Drug in superficial bladder cancer. In: Eardley I, Whelan P, Kirby R, Schaeffer A (Eds.). Drug treatment in urology. Blackwell, Oxford, UK, 2006:176–87.
56. Chester JD, Leahy MG. Systemic therapy for bladder cancer. In: Eardley I, Whelan P, Kirby R, Schaeffer A (Eds.). Drug treatment in urology. Blackwell, Oxford, UK, 2006:188–210.

CHAPTER 10
Prostate Cancer

Ismaila A Mungadi, Olayiwola B Shittu, Abdullahi Abdulwahab-Ahmed

■ INTRODUCTION

Prostate cancer (CaP) is the fourth most common male malignancy. The lifetime risk of developing clinical CaP is 16%.[1] Genetic and environmental factor affect the incidence and mortality from CaP. There is a high incidence among Western and Scandinavian countries, particularly Blacks in America and a low incidence among Japanese and Chinese. There is a worldwide increase in clinical prostate cancer, partly due to increased screening using prostate specific antigen (PSA). Screening has resulted in increased diagnosis of early prostate cancer in middle age (50–59 years), while aggressive radical treatment has reduced mortality from CaP.

The diagnosis of carcinoma of the prostate is made on clinical assessment including digital rectal examination, serum PSA, and transrectal biopsy.

■ ROLE OF MEDICAL TREATMENT

Early detection of CaP offers a chance for cure. Stages 1 and 2 (Table 10.1)[2] are treated by radical prostatectomy; with radiotherapy and cryosurgery as options. Stage T3, T4, and metastatic cancer cannot be cured with radical surgery. For these stages hormonal therapy is palliative and may improve survival.[3,4]

Most prostatic cancer cells are androgen dependent and at least an initial response is expected with androgen deprivation. Withdrawal of androgens leads to apoptosis of CaP cells. Endocrine deprivation can be achieved through various levels of the pituitary-gonadal axis (Table 10.2).

Testosterone, produced by Leydigs cells in the testes constitutes about 90–95% of androgens. The remaining come from zona fasciculata and reticularis of the adrenal cortex. Free testosterone enters prostatic cells by passive diffusion and is converted to dihydrotestosterone (DHT) through the action of and 5α reductase (types 1 and 2). DHT binds to androgen cytoplasmic receptor and the DHT and receptor complex interact with nuclear DNA leading to transcriptional events and protein synthesis. Adrenal androgens,

Table 10.1: Tumor node metastasis (TNM) classification of CaP

T: Primary Tumor	
TX	Primary tumor cannot be assessed
T0	No evidence of primary tumor
T1	Clinically inapparent tumor not palpable or visible by imaging
T1a	Tumor incidental histological in finding 5% or less of tissue resected.
T1b	Tumor incidental histological finding in more than 5% of tissue resected.
T1c	Tumor identified by needle biopsy (e.g., because of elevated PSA level).
T2	Tumor confined within the prostate
T2a	Tumor involves one half of one lobe or less
T2b	Tumor involves more than half of one lobe, but not both lobes
T2c	Tumor involves both lobes
T3	Tumor extends through the prostatic capsule
T3a	Extracapsular extension (unilateral or bilateral)
T3b	Tumor invades seminal vesicle(s)
T4	Tumor fixed or invades adjacent structures other than seminal vesicles: bladder neck, external sphincter, rectum, levator muscles, or pelvic wall.
N: Regional Lymph Nodes	
NX	Regional lymph nodes cannot be assessed
N0	No regional lymph nodes metastasis
N1 Regional Lymph Nodes Metastasis	
M: Distant Metastases	
MX	Distant metastasis cannot be assessed
M0	No distant metastasis
M1	Distant metastasis
M1a	Non-regional lymph node(s)
M1b	Bones(s)
M1c	other site(s)

Source: Sobin LH, Wittekind CH (Eds.). TNM classification of malignant tumors, 6th ed. Wiley-Liss, New York, NY, 2002.

mainly androstenedione and dehydroepiandrosterone, can be metabolized to testosterone and DHT.

Androgen deprivation can be achieved with:
- α-reductase inhibition,
- Androgen blockage using antiandrogen or medical castration using estrogens or luteinizing hormone, releasing hormone agonist and antagonist.

Table 10.2: Medical therapy for prostate cancer

Hormones			
Pituitary:			
LHRH Agonist			
	Buserelin	Sc	500 µg 8 hourly 7 days then intra-nasal
	Goserelin	Sc	10.8 mg 3 monthly or 3.6 mg monthly
	Leuprolide	Im	22.5 mg every 3 months or 7.5 mg monthly
	Leuprorelin	im/sc	3.75 mg monthly or 11.25 mg 3 monthly
	Triptorelin	im/sc	3.75 mg 4 weekly
	Nafarelin	nasal spray	200–400 µg twice daily
Adrenal:			
	Ketoconazole	oral 400 mg daily	
	Aminoglutethimide	oral 250 mg daily	
Prostate:			
	Cyproterone Acetate	oral 200–300 mg daily in 2 divided doses	
	Finasteride	oral 5 mg daily	
	Dutasteride	oral 0.5 mg daily	
	Bicalutamide	oral 50 mg daily	
	Flutamide	250 mg 3 times per day	
	Nilutamide	oral 150 mg daily.	
Chemotherapeutic Agents:			
– Docetaxel			
– Paclitaxel			
– Mitoxantrone			
– Cabazitaxel			
– Abiraterone			
Biophosphonates:			
– Zoledronic acid			
– Pamidronate			
– Etidronate			

The aim of medical castration is to block testicular androgens. A combination of medical castration and antiandrogen targeted to block adrenal androgen constitute maximal androgen blockade.

CaP may become hormone refractory (HRPC) after a median time of 18 months treatment.[5]

Second-line adrenal androgen deprivation using ketoconazole or second-line antiandrogen may be tried. Mitoxantrone a semisynthetic anthracenedione with some structural similarities to doxorubicin has a modest activity and may improve symptoms in HRPC.[6] Paclitaxel, in combination with prednisone every 3 weeks, significantly improves survival in patients with metastatic and HRPC.

Endocrine therapy leads to side effects that represent an accentuation of male climacteron, or andropause. Androgen deprivation leads to reduced libido, erectile dysfunction, muscle wasting, reduced energy, osteoporosis, spontaneous fracture, and anemia. These effects are seen with pure antiandrogen monotherapy.

The future of medical treatment in CaP may be in the development of newer chemotherapeutic agents that can be used as second line in HRPC or as fist-line therapy.

OUTLINE OF PHARMACOTHERAPY FOR PROSTATE CANCER [5–9]

Gonadotropin Releasing Hormone Agonists

Leuprolide, Buserelin, Goserelin, Triptorelin, Nafarelin

Properties: These are synthetic peptide analogs of the natural gonadotropin releasing hormone (GnRH). They exhibit enhanced potency and prolonged duration of action compared to native GnRH. They cause initial stimulation with increased levels of luteinizing hormone (LH) and follicle stimulating hormone (FSH) subsequently followed by inhibition of hormone release. This results in reduced testicular androgen synthesis. When given at intervals of 1–4 hours, they stimulate release of FSH and LH by binding to pituitary receptors. However, with prolonged use, there is receptor desensitization and subsequent inhibition of gonadotropin release. They have been shown to be as effective as diethylstilbesterol combined with bilateral orchiectomy in the treatment of CaP. The half-life of intranasal or subacute GnRH analogs is about 3 hours, with a high affinity to bind to GnRH receptors and a low susceptibility to degradation in the hypothalamus and pituitary.

The long-acting GnRH agonists are used for palliative treatment of hormonally responsive tumors (prostate and breast cancer) and to arrest sexual maturation in children with gonadotropin-dependent precocious puberty.

Side effects: Transient flare of the disease, sexual dysfunction, gynecomastia, hypersensitivity reactions, gastrointestinal and visual disturbances, mood and weight changes, peripheral edema, hair loss, arthralgia, sleep disorders, local irritation at injection site, and depression.

Contraindication: GnRH analogs should not be used for more than 6 months and treatment should not be repeated.

Caution: Care should be taken in patients with metabolic bone disease because reduction in bone mineral density may occur.

Leuprolide

Properties: A synthetic peptide analogs of gonadotropin releasing hormone (GnRH).

Side effects: Transient flare of the disease, sexual dysfunction, gynecomastia, hypersensitivity reactions, gastrointestinal and visual disturbances, mood and weight changes, peripheral edema, hair loss, arthralgia, sleep disorders, local irritation at injection site and depression.

Caution: Reduction in bone mineral density may occur in patients taking Leuprolide. Thus, care is taken in patient with metabolic bone disease. Initial period of treatment may witness worsening of symptoms, the flare phenomenon. To prevent this and risk of cord compression, premedication with anti-androgen is advised.

Dosage: Leuprolide acetate (Lupron) subcutaneous injection 1mg daily, 7.5 mg monthly, 22.5 mg every 3 month, 30 mg every 4 month and 45 mg every 6 month. (Parenteral – 5 mg/ml, also exist as deport suspension – Lupron Depot).

Leuprorelin Acetate

Properties: A synthetic peptide analog of gonadotropin releasing hormone (GnRH).

Side effects: Transient flare of the disease, sexual dysfunction, gynecomastia, hypersensitivity reactions, gastrointestinal and visual disturbances, mood and weight changes, peripheral edema, hair loss, arthralgia, sleep disorders, local irritation at injection site and depression.

Contraindications: In hypersensitivity reaction to any of the constituents

Cautions: Reduction in bone mineral density may occur in patients taking Leuprolide. Thus, care is taken in patient with metabolic bone disease. Initial period of treatment may witness worsening of symptoms, the flare phenomenon. To prevent this and risk of cord compression, premedication with anti-androgen is advised.

Interactions: No known drug interaction with. Its metabolism does not involve Cytochrome *P450* (CYP).

Dosage: 3.75 mg every month or 11.25 mg every 3 month. Leuprorelin can be given subcutaneously or by intramuscular injection (Prostap). Powder for reconstruction is also available.

Buserelin

Properties: A synthetic analog of gonadotropin releasing hormone. It is more potent and longer acting than GnRH.

Side effects: Hearing, sleep, memory and concentration disturbances, anxiety, nausea, vomiting, constipation, diarrhea, breast tenderness, dry eyes and skin, leucorrhea, and leucopenia.

Contraindication: Allergy to its components and hormone refractory tumors.

Cautions: Depression, diabetes, hypertension.

Dosage: Buserelin (suprefact-Aventis Pharma). By subcutaneous injection 500 mcg (0.5 mg) 8 hourly for 7 days, then intranasal spray 200 mcg 6 times daily.

Note: Nasal spray contains 100 mcg/metered spray. Avoid the use of nasal decongestants before and at least 30 minutes after treatment.

Goserelin

Properties: Synthetic long acting GnRH analog.

Side effects: Transient flare of the disease, sexual dysfunction, gynecomastia, hypersensitivity reactions, gastrointestinal and visual disturbances, mood and weight changes, peripheral edema, hair loss, arthralgia, sleep disorders, local irritation at implantation site and depression. Paresthesia and blood pressure changes

Contraindication: Hypersensitivity to GnRH and its analogs.

Dosage: Goserelin (Zoladex) subcutaneous injection into anterior abdominal wall, 3.6 mg every 28 days or 10.8 mg every 12 weeks.

Triptorelin

Properties: Synthetic long acting GnRH analog.

Side effects: Dry mouth, transient changes in blood pressure, gynecomastia, and increased dysuria. Other side effects are same as for Goserelin.

Dosage: Triptorelin IM injection (Decapeptyl) powder for suspension; 3 mg every 4 weeks. Triptorelin as acetate IM (Powder for suspension) 11.25 mg every 3 months.

Gonapeptyl Depot (as acetate) by subcutaneous or deep IM injection 3.75 mg every 4 weeks.

Nafarelin

Properties: Synthetic analog of GnRH. It is rapidly and well absorbed by nasal mucosa.

Side effects: As for Goserelin. Others are acne and rhinitis.

Contraindication: As for other synthetic GnRH analogs.

Dosage: Nafarelin (Synarel, 2 mg/ml 200 mcg/spray), nasal; 200–400 mcg twice daily (one spray in each nostril. Avoid nasal decongestants).

Androgen Receptor Blockers

Cyproterone Acetate, Bicalutamide, Flutamide, Nilutamide

These are compounds that competitively inhibit the actions of androgens at their natural receptors on target organs. They have been used in treatment of advanced CaPs.

A combination therapy involving administration of GnRH agonists and ARblockers (also called antiandrogens) is referred to as complete androgen blockade. This is because both adrenal and gonadal-derived androgens are blocked.

They are divided into two broad groups: The steroidal and the nonsteroidal AR blockers. The steroidal antiandrogens are cyproterone acetate and megestrol, whereas the nonsteroidal include bicalutamide (Casodex), flutamide (Eulexin), and nilutamide (Nilandron).

In clinical practice the nonsteroidal androgen receptor (AR) blockers are more commonly used, they inhibit ligand binding and subsequent translocation of AR from the cytoplasm into the nucleus. They also cause reduction in loss of libido and potency by increasing circulating testosterone levels due to inhibition of testosterone negative feedback at the pituitary hypothalamic axis. However, they are known to cause gynecomastia, mastodynia, vasomotor flushing and varying degrees of decreased libido and potency.

Cyproterone Acetate

Properties: Cyproterone acetate is an effective steroidal antiandrogen and has been found to effectively suppress feedback enhancement of FSH and LH. It has been used in treatment of hirsutism in woman and excessive sexual drive in men.

Side effect: Lassitude, fatigue, breathlessness, weight changes, gynecomastia, changes in hair pattern, rash, osteoporosis, jaundice hepatitis, hepatic failure.

Contraindication: None in prostatic cancer.

Caution: Hepatic impairment, (monitoring of liver function before and during treatment), severe depression, avoid skilled tasks, e.g. driving, monitor adrenocortical function, diabetes mellitus, sickle cell disease (some times contraindicated in these conditions).

Dosage: In cases of initial flare of disease following GnRH agonists or long term therapy, Cyproterone Acetate (Cyprostat), oral 200–300mg/day in 2–3 divided doses.
Then reduced to 200 mg daily in 2–3 divided doses.

Flutamide

Properties: Flutamide is a nonsteroidal potent antiandrogen, a substituted anilide that acts as a competitive blocking agent at ARs. It is primarily used in combination with GnRH analogs in metastatic advanced cancer of the prostate. It is excreted in urine.

Side effects: Nausea, vomiting, increased appetite, galactorrhea, gynecomastia tiredness, insomnia, decreased libido, reduced sperm count, hemolytic anemia rash, hepatic injury, blurred vision, chest pain, and hypertension.

Caution: Hepatic and cardiac disease, avoid excessive alcohol consumption.

Interactions: Enhances anticoagulant effect of coumarins.

Dosage: Flutamide (Eulexin oral tablets) 250 mg 3 times daily.

Bicalutamide

Properties: It is a potent nonsteroidal antiandrogen that appears to have replaced flutamide due to its less hepatic side effects and is taken once daily as against diarrhea 3 times per day. It is used in combination with GnRH with significant reduction in tumor flare. It is also used either alone or as adjunct treatment of locally advanced CaP.

Side effects: Decreased libido, impotence, weight gain, depression, dyspepsia, jaundice, cholestasis, abdominal pain, nausea, vomiting diarrhea, gynecomastia, hematuria, thrombocytopenia, and hypersensitivity reaction (rare).

Contraindications: Hepatic impairment.

Interactions: Enhances anticoagulant effects of coumarins.

Dosage: Bicalutamide (Casodex) oral, 150–200 mg daily as a single agent and 50 mg per day in combination.

Nilutamide

Properties: Nilutamide is a potent nonsteroidal AR blocker recommended for use after surgical castration. It is metabolized extensively into five products out of which one is biologically active. They are all excreted in urine.

Side effects: Appear to be worse compared to Flutamide and Bicalutamide. This includes diarrhea, visual disturbances, allergic pneumonitis and intolerance to alcohol.

Dosage: Nilutamide (Nilandron) 150 mg once daily. However, following surgical castration, Nilutamide is given at 300 mg/day for 30 days and daily dosing subsequently.

Steroid Synthesis Inhibitors
Ketoconazole

Properties: Ketoconazole is primarily used as an imidazole antifungal agent. However, in higher doses than antifungal therapy, it is employed for inhibition of synthesis of steroid hormones such as testosterone and cortisol. It effectively blocks the activity of 17α hydroxylase and 11α hydroxylase in all primary steroidogenic tissues. However, results have not been very encouraging due to associated adrenal insufficiency and hepatotoxicity.

Side effects: Hepatic injury, gynecomastia, oligospermia, photophobia, rised intracranial pressure, etc.

Contraindications: Lactation, hepatic impairment.

Caution: Predisposition to adrenocortical insufficiency; avoid in porphyria and concomitant use with antimalarial drug containing artemether or lumefantrine.

Interaction: Ketoconazole inhibits metabolism of calcium channel blockers, antipsychotics, alfentanil, etc. Its absorption is reduced by antacids, cimetidine, ranitidine.

Dosage: Ketoconazole (Nizoral) 600–800 mg in two divided doses, up to 1,200 mg per day in three divided doses.

5-Alpha Reductase Inhibitors
Finasteride

Properties: Finasteride is a type 1, 5-α reductase inhibitor. It blocks conversion of testosterone to dihydrotestosterone (DHT) in the prostate and external genitalia leading to reduced serum and prostatic levels of DHT. It has a half-life of 8 hours; several months may be required before clinical effect manifests. Finasteride was initially developed for treatment of benign prostatic hyperplasia (BPH), and was found to reduce prostatic volume and improve urinary flow rate and obstructive symptoms. The drug is also licensed for use in male pattern baldness. It reduces serum levels of prostate specific antigen (PSA) and reference range must be adjusted in patients on finasteride. Finasteride is excreted in significant amounts in semen to affect sex partner.

Side effects: Infrequent but include breast tenderness, gynecomastia, decreased libido, impotence, ejaculatory dysfunction, pruritus, and testicular pain.

Contraindications: Children, adolescents, and women of childbearing age.

Caution: Use condom if partner is pregnant or still childbearing, evaluation for prostatic cancer using PSA.

Interaction: No clinically significant interaction reported.

Dosage: Finesteride (Proscar, others) oral—5 mg daily.

Dutasteride

Properties: Type I and 2, 5-α reductase antagonist. It leads to rapid lowering of serum DHT and prostate volume shrinkage than achievable with finasteride. Its clinical efficacy is, however, similar to finasteride and requires several months. Also, excreted in semen to a significant concentration to affect sex partner.

Side effects: Infrequent but include breast tenderness, gynecomastia, decreased libido, impotence, ejaculatory dysfunction, pruritus, and testicular pain.

Contraindications: Severe hepatic dysfunction. See finasteride.

Caution: Use condom if partner is pregnant or still childbearing, evaluation for prostatic cancer using PSA.

Interaction: Serum concentration increased by calcium channel blockers such as verapamil.

Dosage: Dutasteride (Avodart) oral, capsule—0.5 mg daily.

Bisphosphonates

Properties: Bisphosphonates or bisphosphates are analogs of pyrophosphate. They contain two phosphonate groups attached to a central carbon that replaces oxygen in pyrophosphates. They are absorbed onto hydroxyapatite crystals in bone and as such reduce the rate of bone turnover by slowing down their rate of growth and dissolution. They concentrate in sites of active remodeling and directly inhibit bone resorption. Bisphosphonates are very poorly absorbed from the gut, this has affected significantly the bioavailability of the drugs. The bisphosphonates are incorporated into the bone matrix during the process of remodeling and they have the ability to chelate divalent cations. Their antiresorptive activity essentially involves direct osteoclastic apoptosis and inhibition of components of the cholesterol biosynthetic pathway.

They are used in the management of malignancy-associated hypercalcemia and for suppressing the proliferation of cancer-associated proteins. Also used in the treatment of osteoporosis, steroid-induced osteoporosis, Paget's disease and tumor-associated osteolysis.

A modification in the side chain substituents is the basis for their identification as first-, second-, or third-generation bisphosphonates. The first-generation bisphosphonates are the least potent and contain minimally modified side chain. They may cause bone demineralization, for example, medronate, tiludronate, clodronate.

The second-generation (alendronate, pamidronate) carries a nitrogen group in its side chain and these are significantly far more effective than the first-generation drugs. The third-generation bisphosphonates (examples include risedronate and zoledronate) have an attached heterocyclic ring within which is a nitrogen atom and are about 10,000 times more potent than the first generation.

The bisphosphonates are incorporated into the bone matrix during the process of remodeling, and they have the ability to chelate divalent cations.

Side effects: Bisphosphonates cause a wide range of side effects, these include headache, insomnia, drowsiness, nausea, vomiting, anorexia, abdominal pain, constipation, diarrhea, symptomatic hypocalcemia, jaw necrosis, hypertension, etc.

Caution: Take drug with enough water (cup full) following an overnight fast and at least 30 minutes before breakfast. Ensure adequate oral hygiene during and after treatment. In impaired renal and hepatic functions, there is need for dose adjustment.

Contraindication: Severe renal and hepatic impairments.

Interactions: Absorption of bisphosphonates is decreased by calcium salts, oral iron, and antacids, while there is an increased risk of hypocalcemia when given concomitantly with aminoglycosides. Indomethacin may increase bioavailability of tiludronic acid.

Dosages: For hypercalcemia of malignancy by slow intravenous infusion;
   Disodium pamidronate 15–60 mg in single infusion, divided doses over 2–4 days.
   Sodium clodronate 300 mg daily for a maximum of 7–10 days.
   Or single dose infusion of 1.5 g.
   Ibandronic acid 4 mg single infusion.
   Zoledronic acid (Aclasta) IV infusion, 5 mg over 15 minutes as single dose.
   All doses should be tallied with the serum calcium concentration, correct any hypocalcemia before treatment.

Paclitaxel

See Chapter 9.

Docetaxel

See Chapter 9.

REFERENCES

1. Greenlee RT, Hill-Harmon MB, Murray T, Thun M. Cancer statistics, 2001. CA Cancer J Clin. 2001;51:15–36.
2. Sobin LH, Wittekind CH (Eds.). TNM classification of malignant tumours, 6th ed. Wiley-Liss, New York, NY, 2002.
3. Johansson S, Ljunggren E. Prostatic carcinoma cured with hormonal treatment. Scand J Urol Nephrol. 1981;15:331–2.
4. Granfors T, Modig H, Damber JE, et al. Combined orchiectomy and external radiotherapy versus radiotherapy alone for nonmetastatic prostate cancer with or without pelvic lymph node involvement: A prospective randomized study. J Urol. 1998;159:2030–4.
5. Robinson MRG, Smith PH, Richards B, et al. The final analysis of the EORTC Genito-Urinary Group phase III clinical trial (Protocol 30805) comparing orchidectomy, orchidectomy plus cyproterone acetate and low dose stilbestrol in the management of metastatic carcinoma of the prostate. Eur Urol. 1995;28:273–83.
6. Knox JJ, Moore MJ. Chemotherapy in hormone refractory prostate cancer. In: Waxman J (Ed.). Treatment options in urological cancers. Blackwell Science, London, UK, 2002:237–52.
7. British National Formulary. BMJ and RPS, London, UK, 2008;56:363–422.
8. Bhardwa J, Kirby RS. Pharmacotherapy in management of prostate cancer. In: Eardley I, Whelan P, Kirby R, Schaeffer A (Eds). Drug treatment in Urology. Blackwell, Oxford, UK, 2006:161–87.
9. Chabner BA, et al. Chemotherapy of neoplastic diseases. In: Brunton LL, Lazo JS, Parker KL (Eds). Goodman and Gilman's the pharmacological basis of therapeutics, 11th ed. McGraw-Hill, New-York, NY, 2006:1315–1404.

CHAPTER 11
Testicular Cancer

Ismaila A Mungadi, Abdulkadir A Salako

■ INTRODUCTION

Despite its relative rarity, testicular cancer is the most common malignancy in men aged between 20 and 35 years.

Testicular cancer is amenable to surgery, radiotherapy, chemotherapy, or a combination of these depending on the stage and cell type. This has led to dramatic reduction in mortality from testicular tumor over the last three decades.[1] Between 90% and 95% of testicular malignancies are germ cell tumors (GCTs). These GCTs are equally distributed into seminomas and nonseminomas. Up to 60% of testicular cancers have mixed histology.[2] In southwest Nigeria seminomas account for about 15.4% of all testicular tumors.[3]

Several factors contribute to the good prognosis of testicular cancer, once intervention is started early and follow up and surveillance protocols are systematized. Testicular cancer has a predictable channel of spread allowing for precise mapping and surgical extirpation. The stepwise metastatic spread also allows estimation of tumor burden according to the stage. The origin of testicular tumor in germ cells and rapid rate of growth makes it generally sensitive to both radiotherapy and chemotherapy. Testicular tumors are associated with markers that can be accurately estimated thus making early detection of recurrence feasible even before the tumor is clinically or radiologically detectable. This will permit early commencement of chemotherapy on residual and recurrent tumors.

Despite these characteristics, germ cells tumor should ideally be managed in specialized centers because the histology is very complicated and requires expert interpretation.[4,5] Figures 11.1 and 11.2 show early and locally advanced testicular tumors.

■ DIAGNOSIS AND STAGING OF GERM CELL TUMOR

On clinical suspicion of testicular tumor from the history and physical examination, the diagnosis can be established by inguinal orchidectomy.

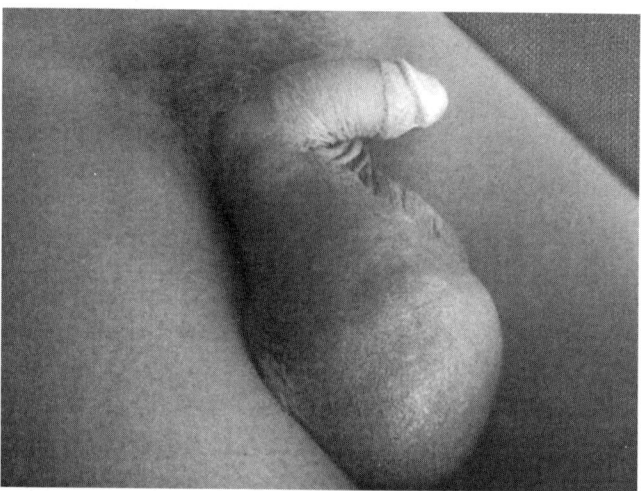

Fig. 11.1: Early testicular tumor in a 24-year old boy with gynecomastia
(*For color version, see plate 2*)

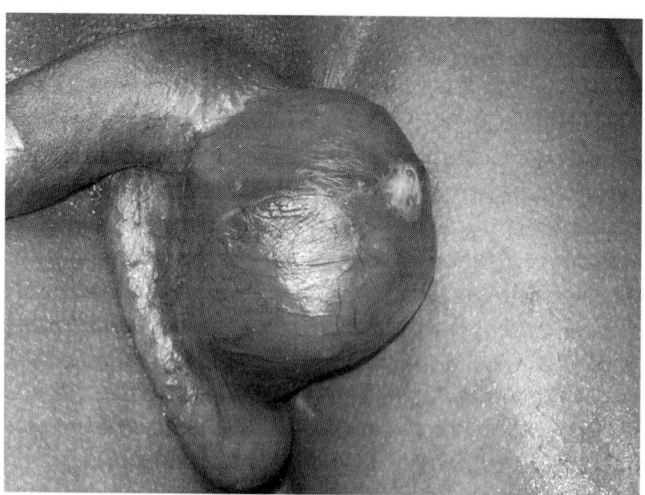

Fig. 11.2: Locally advanced testicular tumor
(*For color version, see plate 2*)

Further therapeutic options will depend on the histologic type, the stage of the disease, and the grade of tumor. The tumor may be histologically a seminoma, nonseminoma (embryonal cell carcinoma, yolk sac tumor, teratoma, or choriocarcinoma) or mixed tumor consisting of more than one cell type, (Table 11.1).

Proper staging will require chest, abdominal, and pelvic computerized scanning (CT) and estimation of serum markers. These markers are alpha-fetoprotein (AFP) beta human chorionic gonadotropin (βhCG), and lactic acid dehydrogenase (LDH).

The staging of testicular tumor is the tumor, node, metastasis, serum marker system (TNMS) system of the American Joint Committee on Cancer

Table 11.1: The recommended pathological classification of testicular tumors by the World Health Organization (from the 2004 version)

1. *Germ Cell Tumors*
   - Intratubular germ cell neoplasia
   - Seminoma (including cases with syncytiotrophoblastic cells)
   - Spermatocytic seminoma (mention if there is sarcomatous component)
   - Embryonal carcinoma
   - Yolk sac tumor
   - Choriocarcinoma
   - Teratoma (mature, immature, with malignant component)
   - Tumors with more than one histological type (specify % of individual components)

2. *Sex Cord/Gonadal Stromal Tumors*
   - Leydig cell tumor
   - Malignant Leydig tumor
   - Sertoli cell tumor
     - Lipid-rich variant
     - Sclerosing
     - Large-cell calcifying
   - Malignant Sertoli cell tumor
   - Granulosa cell tumor
     - Adult type
     - Juvenile type
   - Thecoma/fibroma group of tumors
   - Other sex cord/gonadal stromal tumors
     - Incompletely differentiated
     - Mixed
   - Tumor containing germ cell and sex cord/gonadal stromal (gonadoblastoma)

3. *Miscellaneous Nonspecific Stromal Tumors*
   - Ovarian epithelial tumors
   - Tumors of the collecting ducts and rete testis
   - Tumors (benign and malignant) nonspecific stroma

Source: WHO histological classification of testis tumors In: Ebie Jn, Sauter G, Epstein JL, Sesterhenn IA (Eds). Pathology & Genetics, Tumors of the Urinary System and Male Genital Organs. Lyons: IARC Press, 2004218, 250–262 EBM III.

(AJCC)[6] (Table 11.2). This unique staging incorporates level of serum tumor markers into the staging system.[6]

ROLE OF TUMOR MARKER

Germ cell tumors produce oncofetal protein (AFP, βhCG, and LDH) that are detectable in serum by sensitive radioimmunoassay techniques before the

Table 11.2: TNM classification for testicular cancer

pT	*Primary Tumor*
pTX	Primary tumor cannot be assessed
pT0	No evidence of primary tumor (e.g., histological scar in testis)
pTis	Intratubular germ cell neoplasia (carcinoma in situ)
pT1	Tumor limited to testis and epididymis without vascular/lymphatic invasion: tumor may invade tunica albuginea but not tunica vaginalis
pT2	Tumor limited to testis and epididymis with vascular/lymphatic invasion, or tumor extending through tunical albuginea with involvement of tunical vaginalis
pT3	Tumor invades spermatic cord with or without vascular/lymphatic invasion
pT4	Tumor invades scrotum with or without vascular/lymphatic invasion
N	*Regional Lymph Nodes Clinical*
NX	Regional lymph nodes cannot be assessed
N0	No regional lymph node metastasis
N1	Metastasis with a lymph node mass 2 cm or less in greatest dimension or multiple lymph nodes
N2	Metastasis with a lymph node mass more than 2 cm but not more than 5 cm in greatest dimension, or multiple lymph nodes, any one mass more than 2 cm but not more than 5 cm in greatest dimension
N3	Metastasis with a lymph node mass more than 5 cm in greatest dimension.
pN	*Pathological*
pNX	Regional lymph nodes cannot be assessed
pN0	No regional lymph node metastasis
pN1	Metastasis with a lymph nodes mass 2 cm or less in greatest dimension and 5 or fewer positive nodes, none more than 2 cm in greatest dimension
pN2	Metastasis with a lymph node mass more than 2 cm but not more than 5 cm greatest dimension; or more than 5 nodes positive, not more than 5 cm; or evidence or extranodal extension of tumor
pN3	Metastasis with a lymph node mass more than 5 cm in greatest dimension
M	*Distant Metastasis*
MX	Distant metastasis cannot be assessed
M0	No distant metastasis
M1	Distant metastasis
M1a	Nonregional lymph nodes(s) or lungs
M1b	Other sites
S	*Serum Tumor Markers*
Sx	Serum marker studies not available or not performed
S0	Serum marker study level within normal limits

LDH(U/l)	hCG (mIU/ml)	AFP (ng/ml)	
S1	< 1.5 × N and	< 5,000 and	< 1,000
S2	1.5–10 × N or	5,000–50,000 or	1,000–10,000
S3	> 10 × N 0r	> 50,000 or	> 10,000

Note: N indicates the upper limit of normal for the LDH assay.

tumor is detectable by conventional imaging. AFP is a 70-kD glycoprotein produced by pure embryonal carcinoma, teratocarcinoma, yolk sac tumor, or mixed tumor. It has a half-life of 5–7 days. It is not produced by pure seminoma or choriocarcinoma. Patients with liver disease pancreatic, gastric, and lung cancers may present elevated levels of AFP. All patients with choriocarcinoma and some patients with other GCT produce βhCG.[7] βhCG is a 38 kD glycoprotein with a half-life of 23–36 hours. Hepatocellular, gastric, pancreatic, lung, and bladder tumors and multiple myeloma may lead to elevation at βhCG. LDH is less specific and the enzyme is produced by several tissues including muscles, kidneys, and liver. It tends to correlate with tumor burden and is more useful in assessing advanced disease. The levels of markers are directly proportional to tumor burden and together with the extent of metastasis and tumor bulk, determine the prognosis.[7]

ROLE OF CHEMOTHERAPY IN THE TREATMENT OF TESTICULAR TUMOR

Germ cell testicular tumor may be treated with surgery, radiotherapy, chemotherapy, or a combination of these alternatives. The choice of therapy depends on the TNMS stage, the cellular types, and the prognostic group (Table 11.3), presence of adverse pathologic factors such as vascular or lymphatic invasion and percentage embryonal component.

Seminoma Stage $T_{1-2} N_0 M_0$

The standard treatment is radical inguinal orchidectomy and radiotherapy to the inguinal iliac and para-aortic lymph nodes. The 5-year disease-free survival is 95%. Orchidectomy followed by surveillance and treatment with cisplatin containing combination or radiotherapy if recurrence occurs has resulted in a survival of 99%.[8]

Seminoma Stage $T_{1-2} N_{1-2} M_0$ (Low Volume, Nonbulky)

Radical inguinal orchidectomy followed by radiotherapy to the ipsilateral iliac and para-aortic nodes. This has cure rate of 90%. Also, 90% of patients who have a relapse after radiotherapy can be cured with chemotherapy.[9]

Seminoma $T_{1-2} N_3 M_0$ (Bulky)

Inguinal orchidectomy and primary chemotherapy is the treatment of choice. Radiotherapy is less successful in patients with bulky abdominal mass of greater than 5 cm. The combination in common use are BEP (bleomycin, etoposide, and cisplatin) four courses or EP (Etoposide and Cisplatin) only for four courses in good prognosis patients.[10-12]

Other combination such as VIP (Vinblastine + Ifosfamide + Cisplatin) or EIP (Etoposide + Ifosfamide + Cisplatin) may be used. A 90% 5-year disease-free survival is expected with these regimens.

Seminoma $T_{any} N_3 M_{1-2}$

Inguinal orchidectomy followed by chemotherapy as above.

Nonseminoma $T_{1-2} N_0 M_0$

The standard treatment is radical inguinal orchidectomy followed by either nerve sparing retroperitoneal lymph node (RLN) dissection or surveillance.

In this group the tumor must be carefully analyzed for presence of adverse factors that predict the likelihood of occult metastasis. These are lymphatic or venous invasion, presence of embryonal cell component and the absence of yolk sac element.[13] Relapse rates are high in these patients and may be up to 50%, which can be brought down to only 5% with two adjuvant course of BEP.[14] Therefore, adjuvant chemotherapy may be justified in patients with adverse pathological factors.

Nonseminoma $T_{1-2} N_{1-2} M_0$

Orchidectomy and nerve sparing RPLND if tumor markers are normal. If tumor markers are elevated, systemic chemotherapy should be given followed by surgical resection of any residual metastasis.

Nonseminoma $T_{any} N_3 M_{0-2}$

The recommended treatment is orchidectomy followed by systemic platinum-based chemotherapy. Any residual pulmonary and retroperitoneal tumor can be surgically excised following chemotherapy. Even metastatic nonseminoma is curable with this regimen.

There is an attempt to group patients based on prognostic factors into good, intermediate, and poor prognosis patients (see Table11.3). These groups have a 5-year survival of 92%, 80%, and 48% for good, intermediate, and poor groups respectively.[15]

Good prognosis patient can be treated with three courses of BEP or four courses of EP.

Intermediate prognosis and poor prognosis patients should receive four courses of BEP or VIP or TIP.

Other Uses of Chemotherapy in GCT

1. *Salvage chemotherapy*: For recurrent seminoma and nonseminomatous GCT. Salvage consist of four cycles of standard chemotherapy. Secondary

Table 11.3: Testicular cancer prognostic grouping

Criterion	NSGCT	Seminoma
Good Prognosis Group		
Primary site	Testis/RP	Any
Metastases	No NPVM	No NPVM
AFP	< 1,000	NL
HCG	< 5,000	Any
LDH	< 1.5 × ULN	Any
Intermediate Prognosis Group		
Primary site	Testis/RP	Any
Metastases	No NPVM	No NPVM
AFP	1,000–10,000	NL
HCG	5000–50,000	Any
LDH	> 1.5 to 10 × ULN	Any
Poor Prognosis Group		
Criterion		
Primary site	Mediastinum	No poor prognosis seminoma
Metastasis	NPVM	
AFP	> 10,000	
HCG	> 50,000	
LDH	> 10 × ULN	
Prognosis Based on Risk Group (5-Year Survival)		
Group	Relapse-free Survival (%)	Overall Survival (%)
Good	89	92
Intermediate	75	80
Poor	41	48

(RP = Retroperitoneum NL = Normal, NPVM = Nonpulmonary visceral matastases, ULN = Upper limits of normal, NSGCT = Nonseminomatous germ-cell tumor, AFP = Alpha-fetoprotein, HCG = Human chorionic gonadotropin, LDH = Lactic acid dehydrogenase)

surgery should always be considered where possible in responders, or radiotherapy if surgery is not possible.

2. *Consolidation chemotherapy*: After secondary surgery if viable carcinoma or immature teratoma is found at histology. Patient should receive two cycles of cisplatin-based chemotherapy.

■ OUTLINE OF PHARMACOTHERAPY[16–18]

Cisplatin

See Chapter 9.

Etoposide

Properties: Etoposide is derived from podophyllotoxin, an extract of may-apple (*Podophyllum peltatum*). Etoposide binds to topoisomerace II to form complexes that prevent the binding and interactions of topoisomerace II to DNA, resulting in transcription failure and DNA damage. It is most active against cells in the S and G_2 phases of the cell cycle.

About 50% of the drug is absorbed when taken orally but is usually administered by IV route. It readily becomes bound to albumin, however high plasma bilirubin displaces etoposide from albumin, thus increasing plasma concentration and toxicity of the drug. It is principally excreted via urine, with about 40% being excreted intact in urine. In patients with normal renal status half life is about 6–8 hours.

Indication: It is primarily used in combination with bleomycin and cisplatin to treat testicular cancer.

Side effects: Leukopenia, thrombocytopenia, nausea, vomiting, mucositis, reversible alopecia, allergy, hepatotoxicity.

Precautions: Etoposide should be used with caution in patients with renal and liver impairments, pregnant, and lactating mothers.

Drug interaction: Plasma concentrations of etoposide are reduced by phenobarbitone and phenytoin while it is increased by cyclosporine. Its absorption is also affected by digoxin and phenytoin. It appears to potentiate anticoagulant effect coumarins.

Dosage: The dose of Etoposide when used in combination therapy for testicular cancer is 50–100 mg per square meter for 5 days or 100 ng per square meter on alternate days for 3 doses; however, cycles of therapy could be given in 3–4-week intervals. The continuous IV infusion should be given very slowly over 30–60 minutes to prevent hypotension and bronchospasm due to components used to dissolve the drug.

Preparation: Vial containing etoposide, sodium citrate and dextran as single dose effect agent for intravenous administration.

Ifosfamide

Properties: Ifosfamide is an analog of cyclophosphamide, an alkylating agent.

Ifosfamide undergoes activation by ring hydroxylation in the liver. These produce intermediate reactive complexes from covalent linkages by alkylations of various DNA components leading to disruption and varying degrees of base pair substitution during DNA synthesis. It is this cross-linking of the nucleic acid that leads to malfunctioning of nucleic acids. However, the precise mechanism by which cell death results from DNA damage is unknown. Ifosfamide is for metabolism in the liver. It is given IV. Plasma concentration reaches 3.8 g/m^2–5 g/m^2 and has a half-life of about 15 hours. This varies from patient to patient depending on their hepatic rate of metabolism.

Indication: Combination therapy in germ cell testicular tumors.

Adverse reaction: Ifosfamide causes neurotoxicity, nephrotoxicity, nausea vomiting, anorexia, leukopenia, and myelosuppression.

Contraindication: Hepatic impairments, lactation, and pregnancy.

Drug interaction: Concomitant use with clozapine should be avoided because of the risk of agranulocytosis. Ifosfamide reduce absorption of digoxin and possibly potentiates the coagulant effects of coumarins.

Precaution: To reduce the incidence of ifosfamide neurotoxicity, the drug could be given in IV infusion at a dose of about 1.2 g/m^2/day over 30 minutes for 5 days; patients could also receive IV mesma either as a single concomitant bolus injection at equal dose with ifosfamide or at a dose of 20% ifosfamide dose followed by oral doses 4–6 hours later. Adequate intravenous fluid is also very important.

Dosage: For germ cell testicular tumors (see Table 11.4).

Vinblastine

Properties: It is a vinca alkaloid and antimitotic agent. It is used in combination with bleomycin and cisplatin in curative treatment of advanced testicular tumors. Mechanism of action, metabolism, and precaution are similar to vincristine.

Indication: In combination therapy for germ cell testicular cancer.

Toxic effect: Vinblastine causes leukopenia, neurotoxicity, nausea, vomiting, anorexia, and diarrhea. The syndrome of inappropriate ADH secretion, loss of hair, dermatitis also occur. Cellulitis and phlebitis occur from extravasations during injection.

Drug interaction: The risk of vinblastine toxicity increases with concomitant use with erythromycin and clozapine. Its metabolism is inhibited by posaconazole

Dosage: A curative dose of vinblastine for testicular tumor is 0.3 mg/kg at 3 weeks interval. See Table 11.4.

Bleomycins

They are an important group of DNA-cleaving cytotoxic antibiotics; they are water soluble, basic glycopeptides produced by Streptococcus verticillus.

Table 11.4: Summary of drugs regimens in the treatment of GCT

Regimen	Dose	Administration (Days)	Cycle Duration (Weeks)
EP			3
Etoposide	100 mg/m²	1–5	
Cisplatin	20 mg/m²	1–5	
BEP			3
Bleomycin	30 mg	2, 8, 15	
Etoposide	100 mg/m²	1–5	
Cisplatin	20 mg/m²	1–5	
VIP			3
Vinblastine	0.11 mg l kg	1, 2	
Ifosfomide	1.2 g/m²	1–5	
Cisplatin	20 mg/m²	1–5	
TIP			3
Paclitaxel	250 mg/m²	1 (24 hours continuous infusion)	
Ifosfamide	1.5 g/m²	2–5	
Cisplatin	25 mg/m²	2–5	

Bleomycin interacts with oxygen and fe^{2+} and binds to the amino-terminal peptide of the DNA. This activated complex generates free radicals that are responsible for breakage of the deoxyribose backbone of the DNA chain.

High concentrations are detected in skin and lungs following IV infusion. It is degraded by a specific hydrolase found in various normal tissues including the liver; however, hydrolase activity is low in the skin and lungs contributing to its toxicity at these sites. High plasma concentrations are found in patients with renal impairment, about two third of the drug is normally excreted in urine.

Indication: Testicular cancer, squamous cell carcinoma of the penis.

Side effects: Bleomycin causes significant cutaneous toxicity, including hyperpigmentation, hyperkeratosis, erythema, and ulceration.

These changes begin with tenderness and sweating of the distal digits and progress to erythematous, ulcerating lesions over the elbows, knuckles, and pressure areas. The most serious adverse reaction is progressive pulmonary fibrosis that begin with cough and could be life-threatening; others are hyperthermia, headache, nausea, and vomiting and a peculiar acute fulminante reaction in patent with lymphomas.

Precaution: Doses should be reduced in renal impairment.

Contraindication: Pregnancy, breastfeeding.

Drug interaction: There is increased pulmonary toxicity when used or given with cisplatin, it also reduces absorption of phenytoin and cardiac glycosides (Digoxin tablets). Concomitant use with clozapine increases risk of agranulocytosis.

Dose and administration: It is administered IV, IM, or instilled into the bladder for local treatment of bladder cancer.

Preparation: IV, IM, Inj.

Paclitaxel

See Chapter 9.

REFERENCES

1. Bosl GJ, Motzer RJ: Testicular germ-cell cancer. N Engl J Med. 1997;337:242–53.
2. Mostofi FK: Testicular tumors: epidemiologic, etiologic and pathologic features. Cancer. 1973;32:1186.
3. Salako AA, Onakpoya UU, Osasan SA, Omoniyi-Esan GO. Testicular and para-testicular tumors in south western Nigeria. Afri Health Sc. 2010;10:14–7.
4. Mead GM. Who should manage germ cell tumours of the testes. BJU Intl. 1999; 89:61–7.
5. WHO histological classification of testis tunours In: Ebie Jn, Sauter G, Epstein JL, Sesterhenn IA (Eds). Pathology & Ggenetics, Tumours of the Urinary System and Male Genital Organs. Lyons: IARC Press, 2004218, 250–62 EBM III.
6. Sobin LH. Witteking CH (Eds). UICC: TNM Classification of malignant tumour, 6th edn. Wiley-Liss, New York, NY, 2002.
7. Richie JP, Steele GS. Neoplasm of the testes. In: Walsh PC, Retik AB, Vaughan ED, Wein AJ (Eds). Campbell's Urology, 8th edn. Saunders, Philadelphia, 2002: 2876–919.
8. Milosevic MF, Gospodarowics M, Waarde P. Management of testicular seminoma, semin Surg. Oncol. 1999;17:240–9.
9. Mencel PJ, Motzer RJ, Mazumdar M, et al. Advanced seminoma treatment results, survival, and prognostic factors in 142 patients. J Clin Oncol. 1994;12:120–6.
10. Williams SD, Birch R, Einhorn LH, Irwin L, Greco FA, Loechrer PJ. Treatment of disseminate germ-cell tumours with cisplatin, bleomycin, and either vinblastine or etoposide. N Engl Med. 1987;316:1435–40.
11. Einhorn LH, Williams SD, Loehrer PJ, et al. Evaluation of optimal duration of chemotherapy in favorable-prognosis disseminated germ cell tumours: a Southeasterm Cancer. Study Group protocol. J Clin Oncol. 1989;7:387–91.
12. Bajorin DF, Geller NL, Weisen SF, Bosl GJ. Two-drug therapy in patients with metastatic germ cell tumors. Cancer. 1991; 67: 28–32.
13. Sonneveld DJ, Koops HS, Slijfer DT, Hoekstra HJ. Surgery versus surveillance in stage 1 non-seminoma testicular cancer. Semin Surg Oncol. 1999;230–9.

14. Point J, Albrecht W, Postner G, Sellner F, Angel K, Hotl W. Adjuvant Chemotherapy for high-risk clinical stage I nonseminomatous testicular germ cell cancer: long-term results of prospective trial. J Clin Oncol. 1996;14:441–8.
15. International Germ Cell Cancer Collaborative Group. International germ cell consensus classification: a prognostic factor-based staging system for metastatic germ cell cancers. J Clin Oncol. 1997;15:594–603.
16. Chabner BA, et al. Chemotherapy of malignant diseases. In: Brunton LL, Lazo JS, Parker kL (Eds). Goodman and Gilman's The pharmacological basis of therapeutics, 11th edn. McGraw-Hill, New York, NY. 2006:1315–1404.
17. British National Formulary. BMJ and RPS, London, UK, 2008:56:453–96.
18. Sleijfer DT, Gietema AJ. Testicular cancer. In: Eardley I, Whelan P, Kirby R, Schaeffer A (Eds). Drug treatment in urology. Blackwell, Oxford, UK, 2006:212–33.

CHAPTER

12

Squamous Cell Carcinoma of the Penis

Ismaila A Mungadi, Abdullahi Abdulwahab-Ahmed

■ INTRODUCTION

Penile cancer is a highly tragic tumor. It is a rare malignancy except in some locations in Africa, Asia, and South America.[1]

Squamous cell carcinoma (SCC) of the penis is rare among men who are circumcized in infancy. The incidence of SCC of the penis is decreasing in many countries, probably due to improved personal hygiene.[2]

Human papilloma virus (HPV) and herpes virus infection are strongly associated with SCC of the penis. Premalignant lesions of the penis include leukoplakia, Balanitis xerotica obliterans (lichen sclerosis), Erythroplasia of Queyrat (Bowen's disease) Buschke-Lowenstein tumor (Giant Candylomata), and keratotic balanitis.

Neonatal circumcision, improved hygiene, reduction of HPV, and herpetic infections, avoidance of smoking can reduce incidence of penile cancer.

Penile cancer commonly presents late because the lesion, usually persistent ulcer or sore of the glans or foreskin, is painless (see Figs 12.1 and 12.2). Therefore, delay in seeking medical attention is the rule.

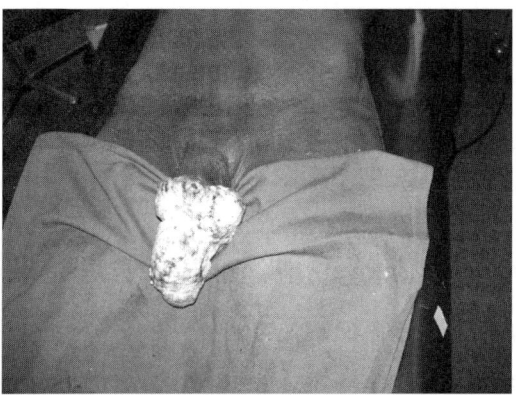

Fig. 12.1: Late penile cancer (*For color version, see plate 3*)

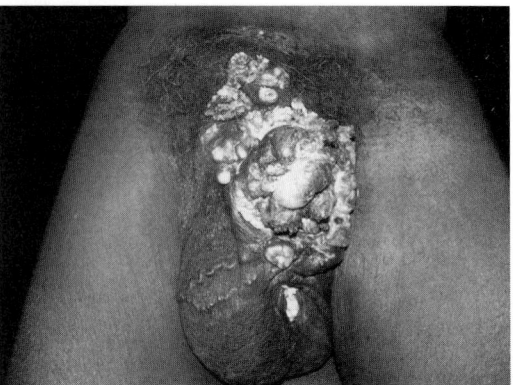

Fig. 12.2: Very late penile cancer
(*For color version, see plate 3*)

The diagnosis of penile cancer is established by biopsy and histological evaluation, including assessment of vascular invasion and depth of local invasion. Ultrasonography, Chest X-ray, CT scan, and MRI may assist in evaluation of pelvic, abdominal, and chest lymph nodes but should not replace careful physical examination for inguinal lymph node. Penile cancer is staged using the TNM staging system (Table 12.1).[3] The Jackson staging was popular and commonly employed (Table 12.2).[4]

The most important prognostic factor in penile cancer is the presence or absence of inguinal metastasis.

■ TREATMENT OF PENILE CANCER

Treatment of Jackson Stage I and II without Inguinal Adenopathy

The standard treatment of primary lesion is partial or total penectomy with 2 cm margin. In Stage I and II, Jackson, the patient, should be followed up with 3–4 monthly examination of inguinal lymph nodes. In patients with adverse pathological factors such as high-grade tumor and vascular invasion, risk-based management of inguinal nodes may be justified. Radiotherapy may allow penile conservation in patients with small tumors.

Treatment of Jackson Stage I and II with Invasion of Corporal Bodies and Tunica Albuginea

Partial or total penectomy with superficial inguinal node dissection. Patients with positive nodes should be offered total lymphodenectomy.

Treatment of Jackson Stage III

A course of antibiotics for 6 weeks should be started immediately following by penectomy and lymphodenectomy.

Squamous Cell Carcinoma of the Penis

Table 12.1: TNM staging of penile tumor

T: Primary Tumor	
TX	Primary tumor cannot be assessed
T0	No evidence of primary tumor
Tis	Carcinoma in situ
Ta	Noninvasive subepithelial connective tissue
T1	Tumor invades corpus spongiosum or cavernosum
T2	Tumor invades urethra or prostate
T4	Tumor invades other adjacent structures
N: Regional Lymph Nodes	
NX	Regional lymph nodes cannot be assessed
N0	No evidence of lymph node metastasis
N1	Metastasis in a single inguinal lymph nodes
N2	Metastasis in multiple of bilateral superficial lymph nodes
N3	Metastasis in deep inguinal or pelvic nodes, unilateral or bilateral
M: Distant Metastases	
MX	Distant metastases cannot be assessed
M0	No evidence of distant metastases
M1	Distant metastases

Source: Sobin LH, Wittekind CH (Eds.). TNM classification of malignant tumours, 6th ed. Wiley-Liss, New York, NY, 2002.

Table 12.2: Jackson staging for GCC of the penis

Stage	Description
1	Confined to glans and prepuce
2	Extends into the shaft of penis
3	Tumor with inguinal metastasis amenable to surgery
4	Inoperable inguinal metastasis, or distant metastasis

Source: Jackson SM. The treatment of carcinoma of the penis. Br J Surg. 1966;53:33–5.

Treatment of Jackson Stage IV

The options are as follows:
1. Palliative radiotherapy
2. Palliative chemotherapy using 5-FU and cisplatin[5] or bleomycin, vincristine, and methotrexate.[6]
3. Multimodality therapy combining neoadjuvant chemotherapy followed by surgery or radiotherapy.

Experiences with drug therapy in patients with penile cancer are limited due to the rarity of the disease.

■ OUTLINE OF DRUG FOR TREATMENT OF PENILE CANCER

Bleomycin
See Chapter 11.

Vincristine
See Chapter 9.

Methotrexate
See Chapter 9.

Cisplatin
See Chapter 9

5-Fluorouracil (5-FU)

Properties: 5-fluorouracil is a pyrimidine analog of the antimetabolite class, (pyrimidine antimetabolites). It is a halogenated pyrimidine. Fluorouracil (5-fu) requires enzymatic conversion by ribosylation and phosphorylation to the nucleotide in order to exert its cytotoxic activity. Several routes are available for the formation of fluoxouridine monophosphate (FUMP). As the triphosphate (FUTP), it may be incorporated into RNA. An alternate reaction sequence crucial for as antineoplastic activity involves reduction of DUDP by ribonucleotide reductase to deoxynucleotide level and formation of fluorodeoxyuridine monophosphate (FDUMP)—potent inhibitor of thymidylate synthesis. This process leads to DNA strand breakage. 5-FU is administered parenterally because of unpredictable and incomplete absorption after ingestion. Metabolic degradation occurs in many tissues, mainly in the liver. It is inactivated by reduction of the pyrimidine ring by dihydropyrimidine dehydrogenase (DPD)-found in the liver, intestinal mucosa, tumor cells, and other tissues. Deficiency or lack of this enzyme causes increased sensitivity and profound toxicity following conventional doses. Plasma clearance is rapid (half-life 10–20 minutes). It enters CSF in minimal amounts. Urinary excretion of single dose given intravenously is equal to 5–10% in 24 hours. Dosages do not have to be modified in patients with hepatic dysfunction because of several extra hepatic degradation sites and vast excess of the enzyme in the liver; it is given by continuous IV infusion for 24–120 hours.

Side effects: These effects may be difficult to anticipate because of their delayed appearance. The earliest symptoms during the cause of therapy are anorexia and nausea, then followed by stomatitis and diarrhea. Mucosal ulceration occurs throughout the GIT leading to fulminant diarrhea, shock, and death, especially in patients who are dihydropyrimidine dehydrogenase (DPD) deficient. Myelosuppression is the major effect of bolus dose regimens. Others are abenua, alopecia, dermatitis, nail changes, atrophy, and increase skin pigmentation, hand-foot syndrome, myelopathy, and chest pain.

Precaution: It is irritant to tissues as such care should be taken while handling the drug. Also to be used with caution in patients with hepatic impairment.

Contraindication: Pregnancy and breastfeeding.

Drug interaction: Metabolism of 5-FU is inhibited by metronidazole and cimetidine with risk of toxicity. Concomitant use with allopurinol, clozapine (antipsychotic) should be avoided.

■ REFERENCES

1. Gloecker-Ries LA, Hankey BF, Edwards BK (Eds). Cancer Statistics Review 1973–1987. In National Cancer Institute, National Institutes of Health Publication No. 90–2789. Bethesda, MD, National Institutes of Health, 1990.
2. Lynch DF Jr., Pettaway CA. Tumors of the penis. In: Walsh PC, Retik AB, Vaughan ED, Wein AJ (Eds). Campbell's Urology, 8th edn, Saunders, Philadelphia, 2002: 2945–82.
3. Sobin LH, Wittekind CH (Eds). TNM Classification of Malignant Tumours, 6th edn. Wiley-Liss, New York, NY, 2002.
4. Jackson SM. The treatment of carcinoma of the penis. Br J Surg. 1966;53:33–5.
5. Fisher HA, Barada JH, Horton J, et al. Neoadjuvant therapy with cisplatin and 5-fluorouracil for stage III squamous cell carcinoma of the penis. [Abstract] J Urol., 1990;143(4 Suppl):A-653, 352A.
6. Pizzocaro G, Piva L. Adjuvant and neoadjuvant vincristine, bleomycin, and methotrexate for inguinal metastases from squamous cell carcinoma of the penis. Acta Oncol. 1988;27:823–4.

CHAPTER 13

Nephroblastoma (Wilms' Tumor)

Christopher S Lukong, Emmanuel A Ameh

■ INTRODUCTION

Nephroblastoma is an embryonal tumor of renal origin. It arises from the primitive renal blastema.

It is the most common intra-abdominal cancer seen in childhood. It represents about 6% of all childhood cancers and accounts for 97% of all tumors of the kidney in children.[1] It usually occurs before 7 years of age, very few occurring between 7 and 12 years and very rarely reported in adults. Approximately 80% of children with this tumor present between 1 and 5 years of age, with a peak incidence at between 3 and 4 years.[2] The incidence of Wilms' tumor presenting in the neonatal period is approximately 0.16%.[3]

Nephroblastoma has been described in the fetus, premature and newborns. The sex incidence is equal.

The etiology of nephroblastoma is unknown, but the disease seems to have a genetic basis. Deletion or mutations in the Wilms' tumor gene (*WT1*) has been implicated. This gene encodes the short-arm of chromosome 11(11p^{13}).[4]

Multiple congenital malformations and syndromes have been associated with nephroblastoma. The most common anomalies are aniridia, hemihypertrophy, and Beckwith-Wiedemann syndrome. The rare anomalies are Denys-Drash syndrome and Perlman syndrome.

In evaluation of this tumor abdominal ultrasound and CT scan are employed to assess the primary tumor. Intravenous urogram may be employed when CT scan is not available.

Largely nephroblastoma is managed according to protocols designed by the National Wilms Tumor Study Group (NWTS)[5] or Societe Internationale d'Oncologie Pediatrique(SIOP) Study Group.[6]

The mainstay of treatment is surgery. Medical treatment and radiotherapy are employed to supplement surgical treatment.

The introduction of systemic chemotherapy to supplement surgery treatment by Faber in 1956 improved survival and outlook of nephroblastoma management. Several drugs have been employed since then for the treatment of this tumor. The combination of drugs will form the basis for discussion in this chapter.

STAGING

Two staging systems are employed namely; NWTS and SIOP.

NWTS-Staging

1. Tumor limited to the kidney and completely excised without rupture or biopsy. Surface of the renal capsule is intact.
2. Tumor extends through the renal capsule, but is completely removed with no microscopic involvement of the margins. Vessels outside the kidney contain tumor. Also placed in Stage II are cases in which the kidney biopsy was performed before resection or "local" spillage of tumor (during resection) is limited to the tumor bed.
3. Residual tumor is confined to the abdomen and not from hematogenous spread. Also included in Stage III are cases with tumor involvement of the abdominal lymph nodes, rupture of the tumor with "diffuse" peritoneal contamination extending beyond the tumor bed, tumor implants, and microscopic or grossly positive resection margins.
4. Hematogenous metastasis at any site
5. Bilateral renal involvement.

SIOP-Staging

1. Tumor limited to the kidney, completely excision.
2. Tumor extending outside the kidney, complete excision:
   - Invasion beyond the capsule, perirenal/perihilar
   - Invasion of the regional lymph nodes
   - Invasion of extrarenal vessels
   - Invasion of ureter
3. Invasion beyond the capsule with incomplete excision:
   - Preoperative or perioperative biopsy
   - Preoperative/perioperative rupture
   - Peritoneal metastases
   - Invasion of para-aortic lymph nodes
   - Incomplete excision.
4. Distant metastases
5. Bilateral renal tumors

TUMOR GRADING

The tumor histology is graded as either favorable or unfavorable.

Favorable tumors are well differentiated, with no anaplasia, while the unfavorable tumors are characterized by anaplasia. Anaplasia could either be focal or diffuse.

■ PRINCIPLES OF TREATMENT AND TREATMENT MODALITIES

The goal of medical treatment or cytotoxic chemotherapy is to maximize tumor kill while maintaining acceptable side effects. The objective is to achieve cure for Stages I and II disease and to prolong disease-free survival as well as symptom free survival for the advanced disease.

The medical treatment as adjuvant therapy is the mainstay of therapy but neoadjuvant may be useful in patients with metastatic disease and in huge localized tumor to control the microscopic metastatic disease and downstage tumor for easy resection respectively.

In this respect adjuvant therapy will be employed for early disease(Stages I and II) and neoadjuvant therapy for advanced disease(Stages III, IV, and V)

Increased understanding of tumor biology and changes in chemotherapy administration schedules has been able to maximize the tumoricidal effects of the drugs.[7,8]

Standard Chemotherapeutic Regimen for Nephroblastoma

The standard drugs used for the treatment of nephroblastoma are vincristine, actinomycin D, doxorubicin and cyclophosphamide. Cyclophosphamide has not however been proven to be any added benefit when used.

The various drug combinations are permutated depending on the stage of the tumor, the histology-favorable or unfavorable, and whether drugs are preoperative(neoadjuvant) or postoperative(adjuvant).[7,8] The various drug combinations are discussed in the relevant sections below.

Preoperative Chemotherapeutic Regimen (Neoadjuvant)

This is employed in advanced disease to down stage tumor mass and also in early disease when it is suspected that occult metastases might have occurred. The drugs used here, are vincristine and actinomycin D. These drugs are administered for a duration of 4 weeks, after which surgery is undertaken. The regimen is elucidated in Table 13.1.

Adjuvant Chemotherapy for Favorable Histology

The two used here, are vincristine and actinomycin D. They are administered for a duration of 18 weeks (Tables 13.2 and 13.3).

Adjuvant Chemotherapy for Unfavorable Histology

This regimen is carefully planned for diffuse anaplastic tumor. Note the various drugs in Table 13.4.

Nephroblastoma (Wilms' Tumor)

Table 13.1: Preoperative cytotoxic chemotherapy

Week	Day	Chemotherapeutic Agent	
1	1	V	A
	2	-	A
	3	-	A
2	1	V	-
3	1	V	A
	2	-	A
	3	-	A
4	1	V	-

Source: Tournade MF, Com-Nougue C, De Kraker J, et al. SIOP 9 Wilms' tumor trial and study results. J Clin Oncol. 2001;19(2); 488–500.

Drug doses: V = Vincristine—1.5 mg/m² IV, A = Actinomycin D—15 mcg/kg IV

Table 13.2: Chemotherapy regimen for stage I and II favorable histology, stage I focal and diffuse anaplasia[7,8]

Week	Chemotherapeutic Agent	
0	A	
1	V_1	
2	V_1	
3	V_1	A
4	V_1	
5	V_1	
6	V_1	A
7	V_1	
8	V_1	
9	V_1	A
10	V_1	
11		
12	V_2	A
13		
14		
15	V_2	A
16		
17		
18	V_2	A

Drug doses:
V_1 = Vincristine—0.025 mg/kg/day for infants < 12 months, 0.05 mg/kg/day for children > 12 months < 30 kg, 1.5 mg/m²/day for children > 30 kg.
V_2 = Vincristine – 0.034 mg/kg/day for infants < 12 months, 0.067 mg/kg/day for children > 12 months < 30 kg, 2.0 mg/m²/day for children > 30 kg.
A = Actinomycin D—0.023 mg/kg/day for infants < 12 months, 0.045 mg/kg/day for children > 12 months < 30 kg, 1.35 mg/m²/day for children > 30 kg.

Table 13.3: Chemotherapy regimen for stage III–IV favorable histology and stage II–IV focal anaplasia[7,8]

Week	Chemotherapeutic Agent	
0		A
1	V_1	
2	V_1	
3	V_1	D
4	V_1	
5	V_1	
6	V_1	A
7	V_1	
8	V_1	
9	V_1	D
10	V_1	
11		
12	V_2	A
13		
14		
15	V_2	D
16		
17		
18	V_2	A
19		
20		
21	V_2	D
22		
23		
24	V_2	A

Drug doses:
V_1 = Vincristine—0.025 mg/kg/day for infants < 12 months, 0.05 mg/kg/day for children > 12 months < 30 kg, 1.5 mg/m²/day for children > 30 kg.
V_2 = Vincristine—0.034 mg/kg/day for infants < 12 months, 0.067 mg/kg/day for children > 12 months < 30kg, 2.0 mg/m²/day for children > 30 kg.
A = Actinomycin D—0.023 mg/kg/day for infants < 12 months, 0.045 mg/kg/day for children > 12 months < 30 kg, 1.35 mg/m²/day for children > 30 kg.
D = Doxorubicin—0.75 mg/kg/day for infants < 12 months, 1.5 mg/kg/day for children > 12 months < 30 kg, 45 mg/m²/day for children > 30 kg.

Table 13.4: Chemotherapeutic regimen for stage II–IV diffuse anaplasia[7,8]

Week	Chemotherapeutic Agent		
0	D		
1			
2	V_1		
3	V_1		
4	C_5	E	
5	V_1		
6	V_1		
7	D	V_1	C_3
8	V_1		
9	V_1		
10	C_5	E	
11	V_1		
12	V_1		
13	D	V_2	C_3
14	V_2		
15			
16	C_5	E	
17			
18			
19	D	V_2	C_3
20			
21			
22	C_5	E	
23			
24			
25	D	V_2	C_3

Drug doses:
The doses for V_1, V_2, D are same as in Table 13.3.
C_3 = Carboplatin—7.35 mg/kg/day × 3 days for infants < 12 months, 14.7 mg/kg/day × 3 days for children > 12 months < 30 kg, 440 mg/m²/day × 3 days for children > 30 kg.
C_5 = Carboplatin—7.35 mg/kg/day × 5 days for infants < 12 months, 14.7 mg/kg/day × 5 days for children > 12 months < 30kg, 440 mg/m²/day × 5 days for children > 30 kg.
E = Etoposide—1.65 mg/kg/day × 5 days for infants < 12 months, 3.3 mg/kg/day × 5 days for children > 12 months < 30 kg, 100 mg/m²/day × 5 days for children > 30 kg.

Chemotherapy for Relapse/ Recurrence

Relapse or recurrence could be a problem with the medical treatment of nephroblastoma. This situation is treated based on risk factors inherent in the patient.

For low-risk relapse, vincristine, doxorubicin, cyclophosphamide, and etoposide are employed for 24 weeks (see regimen in Table 13.4).

For high-risk histology Wilms' tumor, alternating courses of cyclophosphamide plus etoposide and carboplatin plus etoposide for 90 weeks has been found to be useful.

Another modality gaining favor for high-risk recurrence Wilms' tumor is the use of high-dose chemotherapy with autologous stem-cell rescue.

Anti-emesis

The use of cytotoxic chemotherapy may be accompanied by vomiting that could be frustrating. This is even more serious when the patient develops pre-emptive vomiting. It is better to prevent this condition because when it occurs drug treat for the emesis may be abortive. The various drugs used to prevent or treat vomiting include promethazine, chlorpromazine, and ondansetron.

Pharmacokinetics

The pharmacokinetics of various cytotoxic drugs used for the medical treatment have been discussed in other chapters.

Complications/Side Effects of Various Drugs

The complications of the drugs have also been discussed in relevant chapters. It would suffice to say that cyclophosphamide causes alopecia, doxorubicin is cardiotoxic, carboplatin nephrotoxic and vincristine interferes with cellular mitosis.

Recommendations

1. Preoperative cytotoxic chemotherapy should be employed in huge tumors presenting late.
2. The doses for cytotoxic chemotherapy should be reduced to half in infants less than 12 months due relative toxicity in them.
3. Multimodal treatment should be employed with surgery being the mainstay of therapy.

■ REFERENCES

1. Li FP. Cancers in Children. In: Schottenfied D, Fraumeni JF Jr (Eds.). Cancer epidemiology and prevention. Philadelphia, WB Saunders, 1982:1012.
2. Breslow N, Beckwith JB, Ciol M, et al. Age distribution of Wilms tumor: Report from NWTS. Cancer Res. 48:1653–7.
3. Ritchey ML, Azizkhan RG, Beckwith JB et al. Neonatal Wilms tumor. J Pediatr Surg. 1995;30:856–9.

4. Coppes MJ. Haber DA, Grundy PE. Genetics events in the development of Wilms tumor. N Engl J Med. 1994;331:586.
5. D'Angio GJ, Evans AE, et al. Results of the third NWTS Group (NWTS- 3). A preliminary report. Proc Am Assoc Cancer Res. 1984;183:25.
6. Tournade MF, Com-Nougue C, De Kraker J, et al. SIOP 9 Wilms tumor trial and study results. J Clin Oncol. 2001;19(2); 488–500.
7. Grundy PE, Breslow NE, Li S, et al. Loss of heterozygosity for chromosomes 1p and 16q is an adverse prognostic factor in favorable histology Wilms tumor: a report from National Wilms' Tumor Study Group. J Clin Oncol. 2005;23(29): 7312–21.
8. Dome JS, Cotton CA, Perlman EJ, et al. Treatment of anaplastic histology Wilms' tumor: results from fifth National Wilms' Tumor Study. J Clin Oncol. 2006;24(15):1305–9.

APPENDIX

Normal Values* of Some Laboratory Tests of Urological Interest

■ BIOCHEMICAL

Amino acid nitrogen: (S, fasting) 1–5.5 mg/dL (2.2–3.9 mmol/L).

Aminotransferases:
- Aspartate aminotransferase (AST:SGOT): (S) 15–55 IU/L
- Alanine aminotransferase (ALT:SGPT): (S) 10–70 IU/L. Values vary with method used.

Ammonia: (B) 9–33 μmol/L.

Amylase: (S) 80–180 Units/dL (Somogyi). Values will vary with method used.

Antitrypsin: (S) > 180 mg/dL.

Ascorbic acid: (P) 0.4–1.5 mg/dL (23.00–85.33 μmol/L).

Bilirubin: (S) Total, 0.2–1.2 mg/dL (3.5–20.5 μmol/L). Direct conjugated, 0.1–0.4 mg/dL (< 7 μmol/L). Indirect, 0.2–0.7 mg/dL (< 12 μmol/L).

Calcium: (S) 8.5–10.3 mg/dL (2.1–2.6 mmol/L). Varies with albumin.

Chloride: (S or P) 96–106 mEq/L (96–106 mmol/L).

Cholesterol: (S or P) 150–240 mg/dL (3.9–6.2 mmol/L). Varies with age.

Cholesteryl esters: (S) 65–75% of total cholesterol.

Cortisol: (P) 8:00 am, 5–25 mcg/dL (138–690 nmol/L); 8:00 pm, 3–16 mcg/dL (83–441 nmol/L). Newborn, 2–11 mcg/dL (55–304 nmol/L).

Creatine kinase (CK): (S) 10–50 IU/L at 30°C.

Creatine kinase MB fraction: (S) < 40% total CK.

Creatinine: (S or P) 0.7–1.5 mg/dL (62–132 mmol/L).

Epinephrine: (P) Supine < 0.1 mcg/dL (< 0.55 nmol/L).

Erythropoietin: (S) 4–20 IU/L.

Fetoprotein: (S) 0–8.5 ng/mL.

---

*Values are approximate and vary with method used, please confirm from your laboratory

Glucose: (S or P) 65–110 mg/dL (3.6–6.1 nmol/L).

Glutamyl transpeptidase: (S) 8–78 IU/L.

Glycosylated hemoglobin (HbA1c): 20–53 mmol/mol (4–7%).

Lactate dehydrogenase (LDH): (S) 55–140 IU/L.

Lipid fractions: (S or P) Desirable levels; HDL cholesterol, > 40 mg/dL, LDL cholesterol, < 150 mg/dL, VLDL cholesterol, < 40 mg/dL. (To convert to mmol/L, multiply by 0.026)

Lipids, total: (S) 450–1000 mg/dL (4.5–10 g/L).

Norepinephrine: (P) Supine, < 0.5 mcg/L (< 3 nmol/L).

Osmolality: (S) 280–296 mOs/kg water.

Arterial % saturation: 94–100% capacity.

Arterial PO_2 (PaO_2): 80–100 mmHg (10.67–13.33 kPa) sea level). Values varies with age.

Arterial $PaCO_2$: (B, arterial) 35–45 mmHg (4.706kPa).

pH (reaction): (B, arterial) 7.35–7.45 (H 44.7–45.5 nmol/L).

Potassium: (S or P) 3.5–5 mEq/L (3.5–5 mmol/L).

Prostate-specific antigen (PSA): (S) 0–4 ng/mL.

Protein:

- *Total*: (S) 6–8 g/dL: (60–80 g/L).
- *Albumin*: (S) 3.5–5.5 g/dL (35–55 g/L).
- *Globulin*: (S) 2–3.6 g/dL (20–36 g/L).
- *Immunoglobulin*: (S) IgA 78–400 mg/dL, IgG 690–1400 mg/dL, IgM 35–240 mg/dL.
- *Fibrinogen*: (P) 0.2–0.6 g/dL (2–6 g/L).

Prothrombin clotting time: (P) by control. INR, 1–1.4.

Sodium: (S or P) 136–145 mEq/L (136–145 nmol/L)

Specific gravity: (B) 1.056 (varies with temperature, hemoglobin and protein concentration). (S) 1.0254–1.0288 (varies with protein concentration and temperature).

Triglycerides: (S) > 165 mg/dL (1.9 mmol/L) (see Lipid fractions).

Urea nitrogen: (S or P) 8–25 mg/dL (2.9–8.9 mmol/L). Do not use anticoagulant containing ammonium oxalate.

Uric acids: (S or P) Men, 3–9 mg/dL (0.18–0.54 mmol/L); women, 2.5–7.5 mg/dL (0.15–0.45 mmol/L).

Normal Values of Some Laboratory Tests of Urological Interest

■ HEMATOLOGICAL

Bleeding time: Template method, 3–9 min (180–540 s).

Hematocrit (PCV): Men, 40–52%; Women, 37–47%.

Partial thromboplastin time: Activated, 25–37 s.

Platelets: 150,000–400,000/mL (0.15–0.40 × 10^{12}/L).

Prothrombin: INR, 1–1.4.

Sedimentation rate: Less than 20 mm/h (Westergren).

White blood count (leukocytes): 5000–10,000/mL (5–10 × 10^9/L).

■ HORMONES

Adrenal

- *Aldosterone*: (P) Supine, normal salt intake, 2–9 ng/dL (56–250 pmol/L): increased when upright.
- *Cortisol*: (S) 8:00 am, 5–20 mcg/dL (0.14–0.55 mmol/L); 8:00 pm, >10 mcg/dL (> 0.28 mmol/L).
- *Deoxycortisol*: (S) After metyrapone, > 7 mg/dL (> 0.2 mmol/L).
- *Dopamine*: (P) < 135 pg/mL
- *Epinephrine*: (P) < 0.1 ng/mL (< 0.55 nmol/L).
- *Norepinephrine*: (P) < 0.5 mcg/L (< 3 nmol/L).

Catecholamines: (U) Total, 14–110 mcg/24h. Epinephrine, 0.5–20 mcg/24h. Norepinephrine, 15–80 mcg/24h. Metanephrine, 140–785 mcg/24h. Normetanephrine, 75–375 mcg/24h. Values varies with methods used.

Cortisol, free: (U) 20–100 mcg/24h (0.55–2.76 mmol).

11,17-Hydroxycorticoids: (U) Men, 4–12 mg/24 h; Women, 4–8 mg/24 h. Values vary with method used.

17-Ketosteroids: (U) under 8 years, 0–2 mg/24 h; Adolescents, 2–20 mg/24 h. Men, 10–20 mg/24 h; Women, 5–15 mg/24 h. Values vary with method used. (1 mg = 3.5 mmol).

Metanephrine: (U) 1.3 mg/24h (6.6 mmol or 0.05–1.20 mcg/mg creatinine or 0.03–0.69 mmol/mol of creatinine). Values varies with method used.

Vanillylmandelic acid (VMA): (U) Up to 7 mg/24 h (< 35 mmol).

Gonad:
- *Testosterone, free*: (S) Men, 10–30 ng/dL; Women, 0.3–2 ng/dL (1 ng/dL = 0.035 nmol/L).

- *Testosterone, total*: (S) Prepubertal,< 100 ng/dL; adult men, 300–1000 ng/dL; adult women, 20–80 ng/dL (luteal phase, up to 120 ng/dL).
- *Estradiol (E20)*: (S, special handling) Men, 12–34 pg/mL; women menstrual cycle 1–10 days, 24–68 pg/mL; 11–20 days, 50–300 pg/mL; 21–30 days, 73–149 pg/mL (by radioimmunoassay {RIA}) (1 pg/mL = 3.6 pmol/L).
- *Progesterone*: (S) Follicular phase, 0.2–1.5 ng/mL: luteal phase, 6–32 ng/mL; Pregnancy, > 24 ng/mL; men, > 1 ng/ml (by RIA) (1 ng/mL = 3.2 nmol/L.)

Pituitary

Growth hormone (GH): (S) Adults,1–10 ng/ml {46–465 pmol/L (by RIA)}.

Thyroid-stimulating hormone (TSH): (S) < 10 mU/mL.

Follicle-stimulating hormone (FSH): (S) Prepubertal, 2–12 mIU/mL; adult men, 1–15 mIU/mL; adult women, 1–30 mIU/mL: castrate or postmenopausal, 30–200 mIU/mL (by RIA).

Luteinizing hormone (LH): (S) Prepubertal, 2–12 mIU/mL: adult men, 1–15 mIU/mL; adult women, < 30 mIU/mL: castrate or postmenopausal, > 30 mIU/mL.

Corticotropin (ACTH): (P) 6:00–8:00 am, up to 100 pg/mL (22 pmol/L).

Prolactin: (S) 1–25 ng/mL (0.4–10 nmol/L).

Somatomedin C: (P) 0.4–2 U/mL.

Antidiuretic hormone (ADH); vasopressin: (P) Serum osmolarity 285 mOsm/kg, 0–2 pg/mL; > 290 mOsm/kg, 2–12 pg/mL.

■ RENAL FUNCTION

p-Aminohippurate (PAH) clearance (RPF): Men 560–830 mL/min; Women, 490–700 mL/min.

Creatinine Clearance:

Cockcroft and Gault equation

Men: (140-age) × (IBW in kg)/SCR ×72

    IBW = Ideal body weight (men: 50 kg + 2.3 kg/ inch over 5 feet, women: 45.5 kg + 2.3 kg/ inch over 5 feet).

    SCR = Measured serum creatinine

Women: Calculated value × 0.85.

Jelliffe RW Bed side equation

Men: 98 − (0.8 × (age − 20))/SCR × (BSA/1.73 m^2)

        SCR = Serum creatinine in mg/dL
        BSA = Patient's body surface area in m^2

P: Plasma; S: Serum; U: Urine.

Normal Values of Some Laboratory Tests of Urological Interest

Women: Calculated value × 0.9.

Creatinine clearance, endogenous (GFR): Approximates inulin clearance (see below).

Inulin clearance (GFR): Men, 110–150 mL/min; Women, 105–132 mL/min (corrected to 1.73 m² surface area).

Osmolality: 500–850 mOsm/kg water. Wide ranges are normally achievable.

Specific gravity of urine: 1,003–1,030.

Index

Page numbers followed by *f* refer to figure and *t* refer to table

A

Acetaminophen 7
Actinomycosis 20
Acute
    bacterial prostatitis 15
    infection of prostate gland 15
    pyelonephritis 14
    urinary retention 65
Acyclovir 33
Alanine aminotransferase 151
Aldosterone 153
Alpha
    adrenergic antagonist 63
    agonists 57
    fetoprotein 126
American dwarf palm 69
Amino acid nitrogen 151
Aminoglycoside 26
Aminopenicillins 22
Aminotransferases 151
Amitriptyline 11
Ammonia 151
Amoxicillin 22
Amphotericin B 36
Ampicillin 22
Androgen receptor blockers 119
Anemia 38
Angiotensin-converting enzyme inhibitor 8
Antidiuretic hormone 154
Antimicrobial therapy 13
Antitrypsin 151
Anti-tuberculous drugs 29
Arterial
    $PaCO_2$ 152
    PO_2 152
Ascorbic acid 151
Aspartate aminotransferase 151
Asymptomatic inflammatory prostatitis 15
Augmenting citrate excretion 76
Azithromycin 17, 27

B

Bacille Calmette-Guérin 96, 102
Bacterial prostatitis 15
Balanitis xerotica obliterans 137
Benign
    prostatic hyperplasia 62, 121
    urological diseases 1
Benzyl benzoate 35
Beta human chorionic gonadotropin 126
Bicalutamide 119, 120
Bilateral renal tumors 143
Bilirubin 151
Birt Hogg-Dube disease 89
Bisphosphonates 11, 122
Bladder
    cancer 94
    carcinoma 19, 101*f*
Bleomycin 133, 140
Bone disease 70
Botulinum A toxin 59
Bowel disease 71
Bowen's disease 137
Brugia
    malayi 18
    timori 18
Bupivacaine 11
Buschke-Lowenstein tumor 137
Buserelin 116

C

Calcium 151
Candida
    albicans 19
    glabrata 19
    kruzei 19
    parapsilosis 19
    tropicalis 19
Carbamazepine 6
Carboplatin 106
Carcinoma in situ 97

Catecholamines 153
Catheterization 14
Cavernous artery injury 83
Ceftriazone 17
Celecoxib 9
Cephalosporins 25
Chancroid 27
Chemodissolution of stones 74
Chlamydia trachomatis 16
Chloride 151
Cholesterol 151
Cholesteryl esters 151
Choriocarcinoma 127
Chronic
    abacterial prostatitis 15
    bacterial prostatitis 15
    pelvic pain syndrome 5, 15
    urinary schistosomiasis 18
Ciprofloxacin 17
Cisplatin 105, 132, 140
Classification of testicular tumors 127t
Clonazepam 6
Clonorchis sinensis 34
Clostridium difficile 29
Combination therapy 48, 65
Computerized tomographic scan 101f
Consolidation chemotherapy 131
Control of micturition 51
Controlling oxalate excretion 77
Cotrimoxazole 23
Creatine kinase 151
    MB fraction 151
Creatinine 151
Cyproterone acetate 119
Cystectomy 96
Cystine stones 78
Cystinuria 73
Cystitis 15

D

Delequamine 47
Desmopressin acetate 56
Diarrhea 29, 38
Diclofenac 8
    sodium 74
Diethyl carbamazine 19, 34
Dihydrocodeine 9

Dihydropyrimidine dehydrogenase 140, 141
Dihydrotestosterone 62, 113, 121
Diphyllobothrium latum 34
Distant metastases 143
Dopamine 153
Doxazosin 67
Doxorubicin 103
Doxycycline 17, 29
Dry mouth 38
Duplex ultrasound of penile arteries 42
Dutasteride 68, 122
Dynamic infusion cavernosometry or cavernosography 42

E

Embryonal carcinoma 127
Enteric hyperoxaluria 77
Epididymitis 16
Epididymo-orchitis 16
Epinephrine 151, 153
Epirubicin 104
Erectile dysfunction 40
Erythromycin 17, 27
Erythroplasia of Queyrat 137
Erythropoietin 151
Escherichia coli 14, 22
Estrogen therapy 56
Ethambutol 31
Evaluation of
    nephrolithiasis 72
    urinary incontinence patients 52
Exfoliative dermatitis 23

F

Fanconi's syndrome 29
Fasciolopsis buski 34
Fetoprotein 151
Finasteride 68, 121
Fluconazole 38
Fluorodeoxyuridine monophosphate 140
Fluoroquinolones 23
Flutamide 119, 120
Folinic acid 105
Follicle-stimulating hormone 41, 85, 154
Formation of fluoxouridine monophosphate 140

Fournier's gangrene 20
Fungal infection 19

G

Gabapentin 6, 11
Gemcitabine 107
Genital
    chlamydial infection 29
    herpes 18
Genitourinary tuberculosis 16
Gentamicin 26
Germ cell tumors 125, 127
Giant candylomata 137
Glutamyl transpeptidase 152
Glycosylated hemoglobin 152
Gonadal stromal tumors 127
Gonadotropin releasing hormone 116
Gonococcal urethritis 17
Gonorrhoeae 25
Goserelin 116
Gout 71
Gouty diathesis 73, 78
Grading of urothelial cancers 95
Granulosa cell tumor 127
Growth hormone 154
Guanosine monophosphate 44
Gynecomastia 126f

H

Haemolytic strepococci 26
Haemophilus
    ducreyi 17
    influenzae 16
Hepatic
    disorders 38
    toxicity 29
Hereditary
    leiomyomatosis 89
    papillary renal cell carcinoma 89
Hexaminolevulinate 96
Hormonal therapy 44
Hormones 153
Human
    chorionic gonadotropin 131
    papilloma virus 137
Hymenolepsis nana 34
Hypercalciuria 73, 75

Hyperoxaluria 73
Hyperprolactinemia 85
Hyperuricosuria 73
Hyperuricosuric calcium nephrolithiasis 76
Hypocitraturia 73
Hypogonadotrophic hypogonadism 85
Hypomagnesuria 73

I

Ibuprofen 8, 74
Ifosfamide 132
Imidazoles 37
Infertility 84
Inflammatory chronic pelvic pain syndrome 15
Inguinal adenopathy 138
Interferon alpha 91, 99
Interleukin-2 92
International
    index of erectile function 41
    prostate symptom score 63, 64t
    TNM staging system for renal cell carcinoma 90t
Interstitial cystitis 6
Intracavernosal injection of papaverine 83
Intracavernous injection 47
Intratubular germ cell neoplasia 127
Intravenous urography 95
Intravesical
    chemotherapy 96, 99
    immunotherapy 96
    therapy for superficial bladder cancer 96
Invasive bladder cancer 99
Isoniazid 29
Ivermectin 35

J

Jackson staging for GCC of penis 139t

K

Keratotic balanitis 137
Ketoconazole 37, 121
Keyhole limpet hemocyanin 99

L

Lactate dehydrogenase 152
Lactic acid dehydrogenase 126, 131
Large-cell calcifying 127
L-arginine 47
Late penile cancer 137f
Leucopenia 38
Leucovorin calcium 105
Leukemia 83
Leuprolide 116, 117
Leuprorelin acetate 117
Leydig cell tumor 127
Lichen sclerosis 137
Limaprost 47
Lipid fractions 152
Low flow priapism 83
Lower urinary tract symptoms 62
Luteinizing hormone 41, 116, 154
Lymphadenectomy 96
Lymphogranuloma venereum 27, 29

M

Malignant
    Leydig tumor 127
    Sertoli cell tumor 127
Medical
    management of erectile dysfunction 40
    therapy for prostate cancer 115t
    treatment of
        pain 3
        urinary incontinence 51
        urolithiasis 70
Metanephrine 153
Methotrexate 104, 140
Metronidazole 28
Miconazole 37
Mitomycin C 102
Mixed urinary incontinence 51
Modified Thayer-Martin selective agar media 17
Molluscum contagiosum 18
Monoclonal antibody 92
Morphine 9
Mouth discomfort 38
Myasthenia gravis 26
Mycobacterium tuberculosis 16

N

Nafarelin 116, 119
National Wilms tumor study group 142
Nausea 23, 29, 38
Neisseria gonorrhoeae 17
Nephroblastoma 142
NIH classification of prostatitis syndrome 15t
Nilutamide 119, 120
Nitrofurantoin 22
Nocturnal penile tumescence and rigidity 42
Nongonococcal urethritis 17, 27, 29
Noninflammatory chronic pelvic pain syndrome 15
Nonmuscle invasive bladder cancer 97
Nonpulmonary visceral matastases 131
Nonseminomatous germ-cell tumor 131
Nonsteroidal anti-inflammatory drugs 5, 7, 16
Norepinephrine 152, 153

O

Ocular cysticercosis 34
Ofloxacin 17
Opioids 9
Opisthorchis viverrini 34
Oral therapy 44
Osmolality 152, 155
Ovarian epithelial tumors 127
Oxybutinin 58
    hydrochloride 11

P

Paclitaxel 108, 123, 135
Pain pathway 4f
Panecoxib 9
Papaverine 47
Papillary urothelial neoplasms 95
Para-aminobenzoic acid 23
Paracetamol 7
Paragonimus westermani 34
Parasitic infections 34
Partial thromboplastin time 153
Pediculus humanis capitis 36

Index

Pelvic
    floor muscle training 52
    tumor 82
Penile cancer 137, 140
Pentazocine 10
Percutaneous nephrolithotomy 78
Perineal trauma 83
Perioperative antimicrobial prophylaxis 21
Permanent teeth discoloration in children 29
Permethrin 36
Pethidine 10
Peyronie's plaque 41
Phentolamine methylate 47
Phenytoin 6
Phosphodiesterase 40
    type-5 inhibitors 44
Photodynamic therapy 99
Phthirus pubis 36
Piroxicam 8
Pituitary luteinizing hormone 85
Platelet-derived growth factor 91
Podophyllum peltatum 132
Polyethylene glycol 91
Postoperative analgesia 6
Post-prostatectomy incontinence 52
Potassium 152
Praziquantel 34
Prazosin 66
Premature ejaculation 82
Priapism 82, 83
Primary
    hyperoxaluria 77
    syphilis 27, 29
Progesterone 154
Prolactin 154
Prostate
    cancer 113, 116
    specific antigen 113, 121, 152
Protein 152
Prothrombin 153
    clotting time 152
Pseudomembranous colitis 29
Psychosexual therapy 43
Pygeum africanum 69
Pyospermia 85
Pyrazinamide 31

R

Recurrent infection of prostate 15
Regional lymph nodes 128
Renal
    and ureteric colic 5
    cell carcinoma 89
    function 154
    toxicity 29
    tubular acidosis 71
Retinoblastoma 94
Retrograde ejaculation 85
Retroperitoneal lymph node 130
Rifampicin 30
Role of
    chemotherapy in treatment of testicular tumor 129
    medical therapy in infertility 85

S

Salvage chemotherapy 130
Sarcoptes scarbiei 36
Schistosoma haematobium 18, 19f
Scrotal filariasis 18
Sedimentation rate 153
Selective
    cyclooxygenase-2 inhibitors 8
    serotonin reuptake inhibitors 81
Seminoma 127
Serenoa repens 69
Sertoli cell tumor 127
Sex cord 127
Sexually transmitted infections 17
Shock wave lithotripsy 72
Sickle cell disease 83
Sildenafil 45
Silodosin 67
Spermatocytic seminoma 127
Spinal cord injury 83
Squamous cell carcinoma of penis 134, 137
Staphylococcus
    epidermidis 14
    saprophyticus 14
Steroid synthesis inhibitors 121
Steven-Johnson syndrome 23
Streptococcus faecalis 14
Streptomyces nodesus 36
Streptomycin 32
Stress urinary incontinence 51

Struvite stones 78
Superficial bladder cancer 96
Suprapubic aspiration 14
Syncytiotrophoblastic cells 127
Syphilis 17, 29
Systemic chemotherapy 96
    for metastatic disease 100

T

Tadalafil 45
Taenia solium 34
Tamsulosin 68
Tenoxica 8
Teratoma 127
Terazosin 66
Testicular
    cancer 125, 134
        prognostic grouping 131t
        tumor 126f
Tetracycline 28, 29
Thrombocytopenia 38
Thrombocytosis 38
Thyroid-stimulating hormone 154
TNM
    classification for testicular cancer 128t
    staging of
        bladder cancer 95t
        penile tumor 139t
Toxic epidermal necrolysis 23
Transitional cell carcinoma of bladder 103
Transurethral resection of bladder tumor
    96, 97
Trazodone 47
Treatment of
    erectile dysfunction 42
    penile cancer 138
Treponema pallidum 17
Trichomonas vaginalis 28
Tricyclic antidepressants 11, 57
Triglycerides 152
Trimethoprim-sulfamethoxazole 14, 23
Triptorelin 116, 118
Trospium chloride 59
Tuberculosis 16
Tumor
    containing germ cell 127
    grading 143
    node metastasis classification of CaP
        114t
    of collecting ducts and rete testis 127

Tunica albuginea 138
Turulopsis glabrata 19
Tyrosin kinase inhibitors 91, 92

U

Ultrasonography 95
Upper abdominal pain and gastroenteritis
    38
Urea nitrogen 152
Urethelial cancer of bladder 96
Urethritis 17
Urge urinary incontinence 51
Uric acids 152
Urinary
    incontinence 52, 53
    schistosomiasis 18
    tract infection 13, 14t, 52
Urological cancer pain 6
Urtica dioica 69

V

Valproate 6
Vanillylmandelic acid 153
Vardenafil 45
Vascular endothelial growth factor 91
Vasopressin 154
Very late penile cancer 138f
Vincristine 106, 140
Visual analogue scale 4
Vomiting 23, 29, 38
Von Hippel-Lindau disease 89

W

White blood count 153
WHO analgesic ladder 4f
Wilms' tumor 142
    gene 142
Wuchereria bancrofti 18, 19

Y

Yohimbine 47
Yolk sac tumor 127

Z

Zoledronic acid 123